Molton Brown

A WAY OF LOOKING

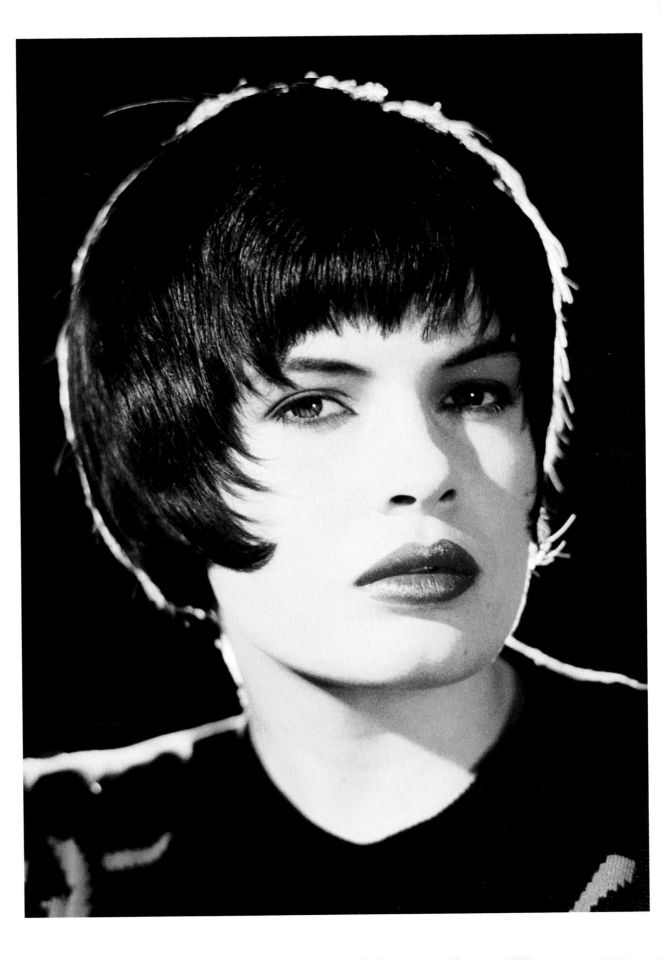

Molton Brown

A WAY OF LOOKING

Lucinda Pearce

GUILD PUBLISHING LONDON

Acknowledgments

All photographs were taken by Richard Lohr except for the following: pages 111, 126, 129, 131, 133, 134 by Aemonn J. McCabe; pages 16, 17, 18 by Sandra Lousada; pages 19, 20, 21 by Simon Bottomley.

Hair by Michael Collis.
Styling by Caroline Collis and Liz Earle.
Make-up by Ariane.

With thanks to Kelly Farmer, Liam Byrne, Sam Darcy and Dale Daxon Bowers.

Clothes from Browns.

Accessories from Butler and Wilson and Studium at Grays Antique Market.

This edition published in 1987 by Book Club Associates by arrangement with Ward Lock Limited, London, and Egmont Company.

CONTENTS

FOREWORD

If you ask me what I think I am, I would say that I am an inventor rather than a hairdresser. I respond best to a need and this is what fires my inventiveness and imagination. This must come from my mother, and my healthy outlook on life must come from my father-in-law. I always look back to one fundamental point which is the way we look at our work and our lives. This is a two-way process and it is all about ways of looking. The woman is looking at herself and at her life; and I am looking at her and at the same time noticing the whole process of my craft. This is why we called our book *A Way of Looking*.

Working in the early '60s I was involved with geometric hair-styles. The emphasis was on the perfect hair-cut and when it worked it was fantastic, but it was very difficult to find the right face to go with the hair-style. In fact one did not even bother to try. If the hair was good enough to take the hair-cut, that was enough. Everyone wanted to have the latest hair-cut and you knew what they were going to ask for even before they spoke. The hair-cut was supposed to make a statement.

However, nothing was individual, except when the hair-cut actually worked, then it was marvellous. Although no one cared whether it worked, they just wanted to have the latest hair-cut.

For many people, hairdressing was still very much about setting, back-combing and spraying the hair to make it stiff. The hairdresser ruled supreme and as a result, many women began to dread a visit to a hair salon. The finished look was created at the expense of the condition of the hair because of heavy-handed use of fierce, hot blow-dryers, harsh tongs and a lot of back combing. I felt more and more ill at ease working in this way. I found that I had a love of long hair, which was something most hair-dressers had no training and no interest in. During training evenings I started experimenting with hair, putting it up without any pins and grips, simply using the hair itself to tie it and hold it in place. While I was practising on long hair I noticed its condition and saw how it reacted to being allowed to dry naturally in its own time. It not only dried quickly but also had a shine and softness to it that could never be achieved with the accepted setting lotions and hair sprays. These discoveries led me in a completely new direction, and were the beginnings that inspired the Molton Brown salon.

I wanted a completely new approach which put all the emphasis on making a woman's hair naturally beautiful. In order to achieve this I found I was not only creating new hair-cutting techniques but also new drying and setting techniques. New ways of setting hair resulted in the invention of a roller called the Molton Browner which was followed a little later by the Molton 'permer', and 'styler'. Perhaps most important of all was the fact that I was offering a service to women by creating a salon where they felt welcomed, comfortable, cared for and confident.

Michael Collis

INTRODUCTION

It is now more than fifteen years since Michael Collis opened Molton Brown and sat waiting for the telephone to ring, hoping that the clients that he had left behind would track him down in his new salon in South Molton Street. The challenge was tremendous. He was opening a new salon, yet he was refusing to backcomb hair or use hairspray. How could he survive with such high ideals?

Michael felt so strongly that what he was doing was right that not only has Molton Brown survived over the past fifteen years, but it has flourished and prospered as its influence has spread. His unique approach puts the emphasis on making hair look naturally beautiful. With this came the techniques of forward cutting and finger drying. New ways of setting the hair were explored and resulted in the invention of a revolutionary roller called the Molton Browner, followed a little later by the Molton 'permer'.

It was the emphasis on not only cutting and styling hair to perfection, but also bringing out its condition, and making it healthy and shiny, that prompted the beginnings of Molton Brown's own range of natural products.

This began with a small hair-care range, using simple herbs which had long been known for their beneficial properties, but not yet used in this way. The first shampoos were made in buckets in the basement of the salon. The preparation of the products was uncompromising: only the best ingredients were used and the method of production was laborious. However, at the end of the day Molton Brown had a hair-care line to be reckoned with.

Now, fifteen years on, Molton Brown Cosmetics has not only a range of products for hair care, but also for bath care, sun care and skin care. In addition, it has a unique selection of coloured cosmetics, a collection of perfumes and even pot pourris. They are all formulated in Molton Brown laboratories and manufactured in the company factory which is housed on a farm in Essex. This makes it possible to ensure that standards are kept high and products remain pure. The utmost care is taken to choose only the purest grades of raw materials. Compromises are never made, since only the best will do. Our aim is to create products of the highest quality which are effective and which look, feel and smell luxurious. They should awaken the senses and give you a greater feeling of well-being.

In their work and in *A Way of Looking*, Molton Brown's central concern is the beauty of women. Although external beauty is subjective, we are all affected by our individual perception of it and marvel when we see it. Beauty inspires a feeling of wonder, whether it be a young child in its innocence, a flower in all its delicacy or any one of the marvels of nature.

However, external beauty is not Molton Brown's exclusive interest. Here, the aim is not only to share with you some inspirational hair-styling and wonderful make-up techniques, but also to try and include you in a search which, for Molton Brown, is fascinating – the search for inner beauty and harmony.

A Way of Looking incorporates the thoughts of a selection of people who use healing techniques both in their lives and in their work. Each of them has offered a personal viewpoint on the way to health. From their ideas it becomes clear that no matter what method you choose to follow, if it is natural, it will provide inner harmony and the basis for naturally beautiful looks.

We would like to thank all the people who have contributed to this book, and in particular our special thanks go to Richard Lohr for photography and to Ariane for the generous way in which she has shared her professional knowledge and expertise.

MIMI

◇ Mimi's hair vibrates with a subtle and translucent quality. It was cut to shoulder length which enhances and softens the jaw-line. The fringe is cut very square to widen and open her face. Mimi's hair is not naturally sleek, the shine is achieved by the hair being blow dried then set on very large rollers. These are left in for fifteen minutes

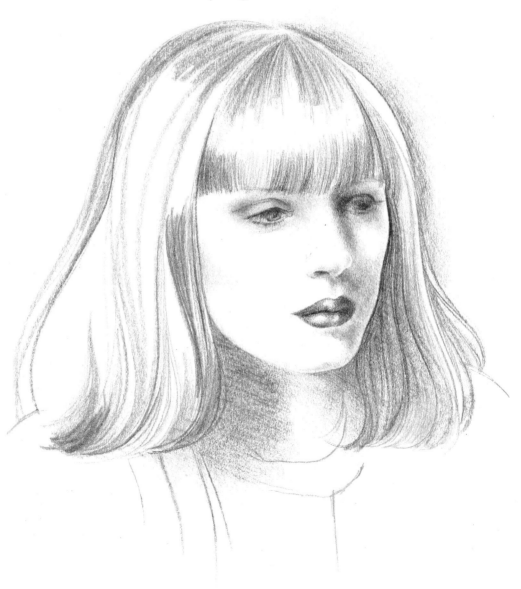

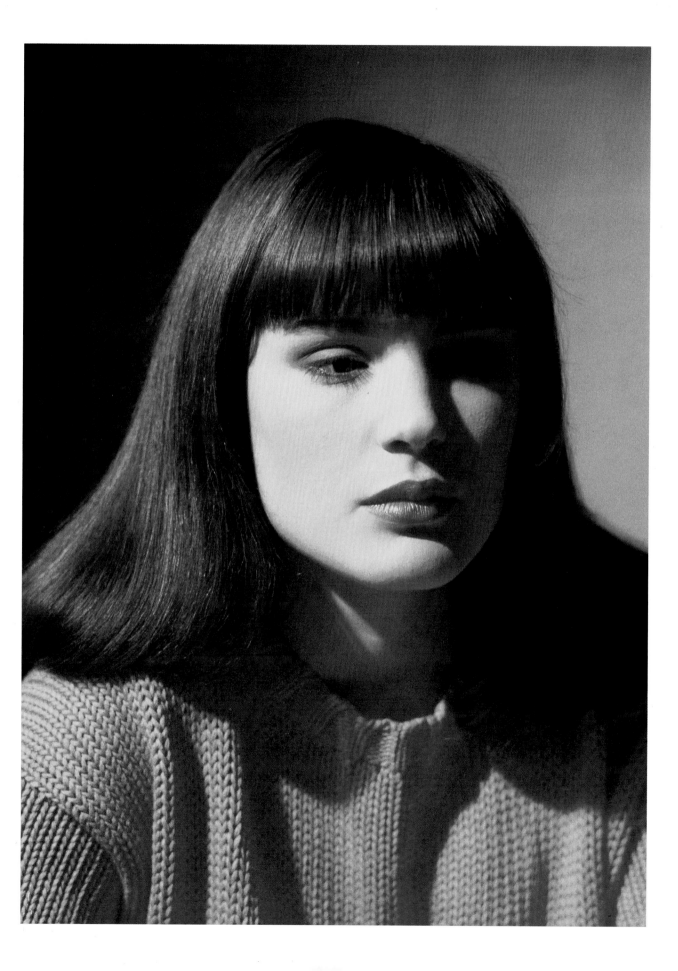

without any heat directed on to the hair. This is a good method for hiding all the little split ends and leaving the hair looking wonderfully sleek.

○ We began by using a light-weight foundation to match Mimi's natural skin-tone. Then, loose powder was lightly brushed over the face in order to set the foundation and to help make the blending of the eye shadows and the blusher easier. The eyebrows were gently filled in, then brushed into a flattering shape.

A pale peach eye shadow was brushed all over the eye from the brow to the eyelash base. Next, a deeper shade of apricot was dusted over the lower lid, starting from the inner corner and continuing to the outer corner. A soft fawn shade was used in the eye socket and blended upwards so that no lines showed. A mid-brown eye shadow was dampened and used as a fine eye liner across the base of the top lash and then blended with a fawn shade to soften it. For the final touch, a rich brown mascara was applied to the lashes.

On the cheeks we used nearly-nude powder blusher, to add shape rather than colour. Lastly, on the lips we see a splash of raspberry-peach lipstick.

Thick, Frizzy Hair

WASHING AND DRYING

Thick, frizzy hair needs washing every few days because the sheer length and weight of the hair makes the scalp oily, although the hair itself is very dry. It needs to be conditioned very well every time it is washed with a medium to heavy conditioner. This hair is very wiry and porous and if it is worn long and it is not layered, it can look wild. Another way of lessening the frizz is to set the blow-dried hair on very large rollers.

Medium-length hair will need washing less often, perhaps every four or five days, because it does not get greasy. It is best to dry short hair with the hands in order to retain the natural oils in the hair.

CUTTING

If long hair is left all one length then it needs very careful setting. If it is graduated to the right length then some of the natural bounce can be used. However, the hair around the hairline is the frizziest and finest and great care must be taken when cutting it. Medium length hair will shrink up when it is cut but will retain its heavy weight, so care must be taken that the cut is just the right length. If thick, frizzy hair is cut really short it can look striking (see Denise).

SETTING
This hair takes to a set very quickly. Unless a woman has very fine features and you want to give volume to the face the hair should be set very lightly. If you set medium-length hair lightly then it will not appear so thick and voluminous. With short hair it is not necessary to set the hair except perhaps at the sides, where it may be frizzy or curly.

HIGHLIGHTING AND TINTING
Tinting and highlights should be kept light and subtle.

General Hair Care

WASHING HAIR
The most important thing to remember when washing hair is to rinse off the shampoo thoroughly. Dull hair and many scalp irritations are caused simply by not rinsing the hair thoroughly. Although everybody has their own individual way of washing their hair, there are two basic methods: one is to give the scalp a good massage, using a circular motion with the fingers; the other is to shampoo the hair in one direction only, from the roots to the ends. The advantage of this system is that the hair is far less inclined to knot or tangle.

When you are washing your own hair, notice how your hair and scalp react to the shampoo you use, both immediately after you have washed your hair as well as on the next day. There are no rules about how often you should wash your hair, because everybody's hair is different. Use a little conditioner on the ends of your hair, but be careful not to over condition it as this can make it look limp and greasy.

DRYING HAIR

Today most people use a blow drier and do not even consider finger drying and towel drying as methods of drying hair. These techniques, although not generally recognized, are both practical and successful.

Towel drying must be done in a systematic way. Take a towel and firmly stroke the hair dry, following the direction of the hair. Keep moving the towel through your hand so that you are always using a part that is dry. (It is often necessary to use as many as three towels to completely dry the hair.)

By using this method, you are working with the direction in which the hair grows and not irritating the scalp. It is amazing how quickly the hair dries and how shiny it appears.

Finger drying once the initial surplus moisture is removed with the towel, use your hands to lift, roll, and turn the hair in the areas where you want height and width.

From time to time, it is a good idea to stop and comb the hair through to check that the hair is drying evenly all over. For this it is best to use a large-tooth comb, as a narrow one may catch and pull the hair.

Once you have mastered the technique, finger drying is easy.

General Skin Care

A proper skin-care routine is essential no matter what skin type you have. But before even talking about what you might put on your skin, remember that the best way to help yourself is by following a balanced diet and taking regular exercise.

A daily skin-care routine will help your skin look at its best. It should be done night and morning and need take no longer than five minutes. At night, it is essential to remove all your make-up and daily grime, so that you sleep with a cleansed and moisturized face.

Start the routine with a cleanser, and follow it with a wash which will remove any traces of the cleanser. Next, use a toner to stimulate the blood circulation. This will also bring any waste material to the surface. Finally use a moisturizer to replace your skin's lost moisture.

In the morning, toning and moisturizing will suffice, as long as you have completed the cleansing routine the night before. Depending on your skin type, a once-a-week or once-a-month, extra-deep cleanse — a facial scrub followed by steaming and a mask — is a great pick-me-up.

When choosing your products, find out what ingredients have been used, and ask whether any colouring or fragrance has been added and whether testing was carried out on animals.

CLEANSE

There are different kinds of cleansers to choose from. Creamy cleansers or cleansing milks are emulsifiers which, when put on the face, clean away make-up and cut through any surface dirt which lies on the face. You can apply these cleansers either using your finger-tips — make small circular movements all over your face and then tissue off — or, alternatively, you can use a flannel, a face brush or a slightly abrasive sponge. Those who like the idea of soap and water and feel unclean without it, should follow the cream cleanser with a facial wash or a special soap. Do not use perfumed soaps on your face as these can cause skin reactions.

WASH

However thoroughly you wipe away the cleanser using a tissue, some amount of residue will always be left on the surface of the skin. If this is not properly removed it will lie in the pores and cause blackheads and other skin blemishes. By washing the face after cleansing, remaining traces of any residue will be gently dissolved leaving the skin feeling soft, clean and fresh.

A facial wash is a thick, gel-like liquid which is rich and creamy in texture. Many people continue to worry about washing their face, particularly if their skin is naturally dry, but some washes are suitable for all skin types. The rich, foamy lather gently cleans the skin without drying, and leaves your face with a bright glow.

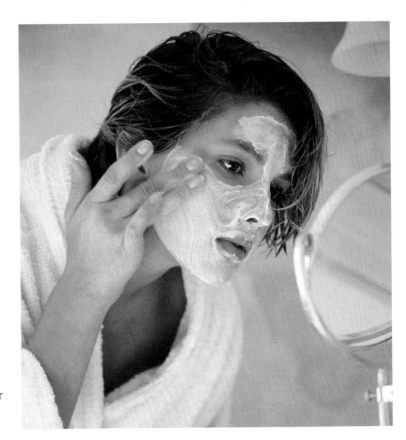

Work in creamy cleanser
with finger-tips and
remove with a tissue.

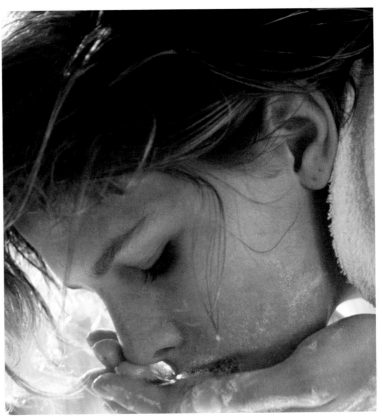

Wash with water and
facial wash.

TONE

A toner accelerates blood circulation and, in doing so, both increases the oxygen supply to the skin and expels carbon dioxide and waste from deep within it. In other words, it will awaken and activate the skin, making it work more efficiently.

All skin will benefit from a toner and there are different ones for every type of skin. For sensitive or dry skin it is best to use an alcohol-free toner. Normal skin does not need alcohol either, although a little in the toner will do it no harm. A small amount of alcohol for oily skin can be very helpful as it helps to blot excess sebum on skin that has over active sebacious glands. The danger with toners for oily skin is that they tend to be too harsh.

Some toners contain a special selection of steeped herbs and floral waters which are in themselves astringent and healing. For oily skin, the steeped herbs clear the skin, while skin softeners in the toner help to prevent flaky skin which, if allowed to accumulate, restricts the flow of sebum and causes breakout.

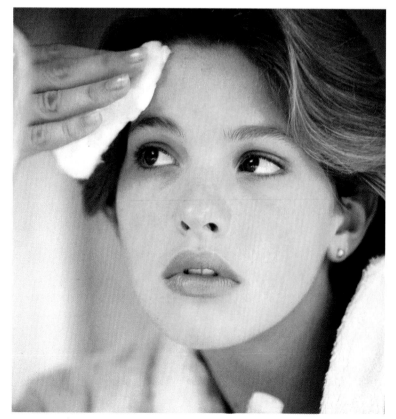

Apply toner with damp cotton-wool to remove any residue.

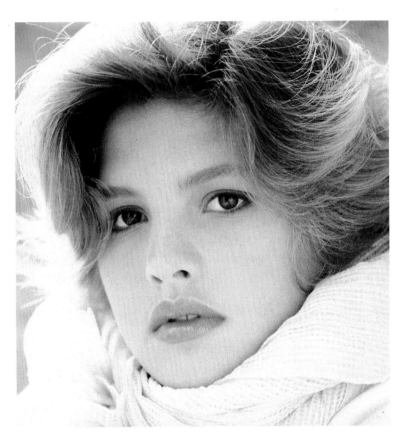

Protect the skin with a moisture retainer followed by a moisturizer suitable for your skin type.

MOISTURIZE AND PROTECT

Moisturizing creams are designed to protect dry skin by coating the external surface, making it feel smoother instantly. Because the skin is then occluded, moisture builds up within the skin and hence it is described as 'moisturized'. The best occluder would be something like petroleum jelly but this would not be aesthetically pleasing, so creams are used instead. Moisturizing is essential for every skin, whether it is normal, dry or oily.

Normal and dry skins need a rich moisturizer although it is not necessary to use a heavier cream at night. Whatever cream you use, it should be gently massaged all over your face and continued down the neck. The neck is often the most neglected part of the body and tends to be one of the first areas to show signs of age. It is also advisable to use a good-quality eye cream. This lubricates and tones the area around the eye.

Even if your skin is oily it still needs moisture, so use a water-based, oil-free moisturizer. It is lack of moisture that causes skin to wrinkle and for this reason a special product called a 'moisture retainer' is now available. As the skin ages, and because of environmental conditions, the level of natural moisturizing fluids is depleted and the skin becomes dry. Natural moisturizing fluids are a blend of sugars and amino acids which 'hold on' to the water within the skin and, in doing so, make it elastic, supple and moist. The moisture retainer is a blend of sugar and amino acids which has been specially formulated to replace the natural moisturizing fluids. Daily use helps to replenish nature's loss to give deep-down moisturization.

SCRUB

This is a weekly, or monthly, routine which supplements your daily skin care. A scrub contains minute grains which gently slough away dead, flaky skin and loosen any impurities which may be clogging the pores. This part of the cleansing routine gives your skin a gentle boost leaving your face with a deep clean glow. Those with sensitive, dry skin may also use a scrub, but should limit its application to the nose, chin and forehead.

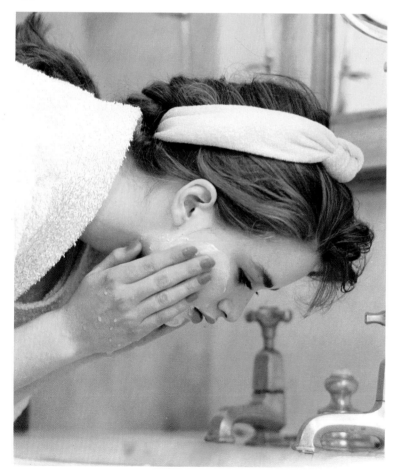

Gently massage the scrub all over your clean face, avoiding the eyes.

STEAM

Steaming dilates the pores, relaxes muscular tissue, and flushes toxins from the skin leaving it ultra clean. Herbal sachets may be put in the water. There are different herbal combinations for the different skin types. For normal to dry and sensitive skins, the ingredients used are clover, comfrey, cowslip, violet, pansy, parsley, lavender, licorice, orange blossom, oil of rose, oil of geranium and oil of cypress. For normal to oily and combination skins, the ingredients used are peppermint, parsley, lavender, lemon peel, licorice, comfrey, hazel, fennel, rose and oil of lemon grass. Cleanse your face before steaming, then cover the head with a towel and breathe in the herbal vapours until the water cools. By this time the pores are fully open. (You might like to soak a little cotton wool in the cooled water and put pads over your eyes to relax and refresh them.) Finally, rinse your face, first in warm, and then in cool, water.

Steam your face over a bowl of hot water for no more than three minutes.

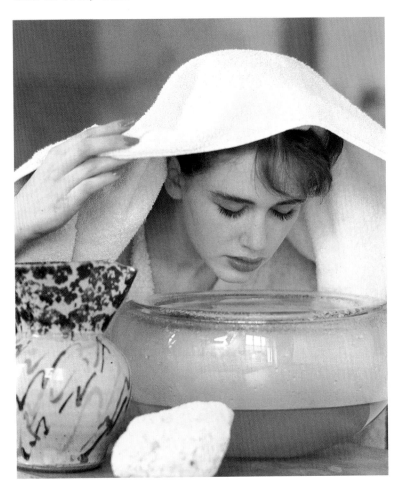

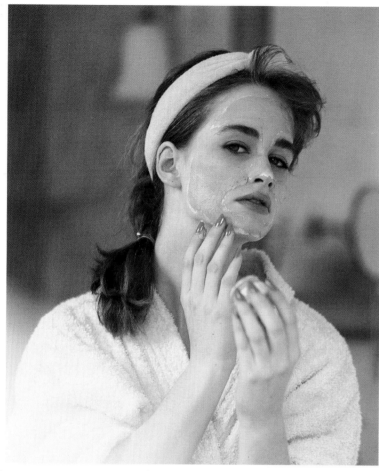

Apply the mask all over your face, avoiding the eyes and lips and relax for five to ten minutes. Rinse off with luke-warm water.

MASK

A mask is more effective if the skin is prepared by steaming. However, it is possible to use a mask without this step as long as the skin has been thoroughly cleansed.

There are different types of masks containing different blends of clays. The clays have strong drawing properties which enable them to cleanse the pores deeply. Some masks contain floral water which softens, tones and revitalizes the skin leaving it feeling firmer, glowing, fresh and moist.

A clay mask is primarily for use on oily or problem skin, but those with dry, normal or sensitive skin may also benefit from it.

Apply the mask evenly onto cleansed skin avoiding the eyes and lips. Leave until dry and wash off with warm water.

Bath Care

Bathing has been an important feature of our lives for many centuries. In the early days, natural hot springs were used to provide soothing, refreshing, and cleansing baths. From the Middle East comes the Turkish bath, from Japan the communal family bath, and from Finland, the hot, dry sauna. The most popular of these in the West is the sauna, which is now a familiar addition to many health clubs. It is unfortunate that there are so few Turkish baths as they are both enjoyable and beneficial. The Turkish bath provides hot steam to open the pores, dry heat to make you sweat, a body scrub (to remove the surface layer of dirt and dead skin cells as well as the acidity build-up which clogs up our pores) and finally, an ice-cold plunge followed by a lovely hot cup of tea drunk wrapped up in a warm towel while relaxing on a comfortable bed. It is hardly surprising that many Arab women visit a Turkish bath every week.

The sauna is more popular because of its practicality and convenience. The dry heat opens your pores and allows you to sweat. It is very important to take a good loofah or rough flannel into the sauna and really work over your body to remove all the dead skin cells. You will be amazed at just how much grime and dead skin can be removed from your body, even though you take a daily bath at home.

The most hygienic way of washing at home is to take a shower. However, although they are becoming increasingly popular only a few people have one in their own home. The attractions of a shower are that it saves time and is more invigorating than lying in a bath. In a bath what you are really doing is soaking in your own dirty water. Nonetheless, it is pleasant to lie in a hot bath because it relaxes the muscles, eases physical tension and provides a little time to unwind. If you enjoy having a bath, try to end your bath-time by splashing yourself with clean water, either using a bowl or a small hand shower.

There is a wonderful choice of bathcare accessories to choose from, starting with the simple flannel, scrubbing brush and pumice, and going right through to natural loofahs which come in every conceivable shape, form and finish. Last but not least, is the most luxurious item of all, the natural sea sponge which, although expensive, is well worth the investment. A word of warning: whatever sponge, flannel or loofah you use, rinse it thoroughly with clean water and wring it out after use. This will help to keep it clean as well as preserving its life span.

There is no end to the variety of fragrances and products which you can add to the bath and shower for a taste of luxury. Products come in an enormous variety of tempting packages. But be warned; many fragrances are highly irritant and can cause more harm than good. There are four categories of bath products:

OILS
Bath oils are often called milks because of their emulsifying properties.

FOAM BATHS
The pleasant sensation of lazing in millions of bubbles is truly luxurious, provided that you buy a good-quality product which has added moisturizers and oils, which will prevent dryness.

SALTS
In general, bath salts can be rather coarse and you may be sorely disappointed when you sprinkle them in your bath. If you use natural salts which have been combined with other sea minerals you will give your muscles and skin a really good boost thanks to the presence of sulphur and zinc.

HERB BATHS
You can have a lot of fun making a herb bath yourself. Try filling a muslin bag with your own choice of natural herbs, or a mixture of rosemary, chamomile and mint. If you are feeling cold and shivery try adding a tablespoon of powdered ginger to the bath.

After a bath or shower it is important to seal in the moisture by using a good body lotion or body oil, both of which will help keep your skin smooth, soft and silky. Products which take care of your body and your skin should be just as important as your make-up and clothes.

Hand and Foot Care

The benefits of taking care of such well-used parts of the body as the hands and feet cannot be over-emphasized. A regular manicure and pedicure can be a pleasurable part of your beauty routine if you follow these guidelines.

MANICURE

● Soak your hands in water containing a drop of Magnolia Bath Milk, or any other mild soapy solution for cleaning and softening the cuticle. Now dry your hands and file the nails with an emery-board (see fig a), keeping

a)
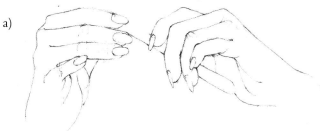

the shape straight across the top. Do not file the nail too much at either side as this will weaken it.

● Paint on cuticle remover and gently push back the cuticle (see fig b) and clean under the nail. Rinse off the cuticle remover and dry your nails and hands thoroughly, gently pushing back the cuticle with the towel as you do so.

● Remove any rough edges with an emery-board. Once your hands are smooth, massage them with a moisturizing hand lotion. Now remove the residue of hand lotion from your nails, either by placing them in warm water and then drying them, or by using a small amount of nail polish remover on some cotton wool to wipe each nail clean.

● Apply base coat to your nails (see fig c), and follow this with coloured nail polish, allowing each coat to dry before applying the next one. You can add a final top coat to give your colour that extra bit of protection.

● If your nails and hands are very dry, this is a perfect opportunity to give yourself a lovely hand massage with warm Vitamin E oil or any rich hand cream. Another wonderful treatment is to dip your hands into warm paraffin wax which leaves the skin clean and beautifully soft.

b)

c)

PEDICURE

● Soak your feet in a bowl of warm, soapy water. A foam bath, such as Bubbling Orange Grove, would be perfect. When you are ready, take out one foot and dry it well. Remove any nail polish and check the whole foot for dry skin or any infection.

● Now file your nails; keep the shape more or less straight across the toes and do not file down the side of the nail. Apply cuticle remover around the cuticle and under the nail. Take an orange stick, covered with cotton wool and dampened in water, and gently push back the cuticle. Then clean under the nail. Now rub away any hard skin under the foot and round the toes with a file or pumice. Replace your foot in the water and, taking the other one, follow the same procedure.

● Go back to the first foot and dry it thoroughly, pushing back the cuticle with a towel. Make sure it is completely dry, taking special care between the toes. At this point it is worth checking the nail edges again with an emery-board. Remove any loose cuticle with nail clippers, working carefully round the nail without actually cutting the cuticle itself. Then put cream on your foot and massage it with long, sweeping strokes, using a hand cream or a light oil such as Orange Body Oil.

● Clean your nails with a little nail polish remover on a piece of cotton wool. This removes any cream left over from the massage. Next space out your toes using cotton-wool which has been rolled, twisted, and then threaded between the toes.

● Apply the base coat; which acts as a protection and provides a good surface for the enamel. Apply two coats of enamel and then add a final top coat for that extra finish.

● Take the other foot and follow the second half of the routine to the end.

AROMATHERAPY

I try to maintain good health and balance by being aware of the needs of my body, by cultivating regular living habits, by making time for rest and relaxation and by getting out in the fresh air as much as possible. To maintain a balanced inner life means being aware of my inner needs. Breathing and meditation as well as physical exercises all contribute towards achieving this.

In the morning before rising, try some simple leg exercises. Lie on your back and move your legs, bicycle fashion. Start slowly. In order to unlock energy in the morning, I do warm-up exercises which help to get me, and my energy, moving. They also help to improve the articulation of the joints. You might choose to study tai-chi or yoga, which are forms of exercises which establish a link between body and mind.

Food is a basic need of the body and the quality of it is important. I try to avoid chemicals, preservatives and colourings while ensuring that I take plenty of fresh foods — fruit, salads and vegetables. I try to eat natural, unrefined foods where possible. Finally, I am careful with my choice of food and avoid, for example, greasy food which can cause bad skin. The human body can be compared to a car engine — the better the grade of petrol the better the performance of the engine!

The essence of well-being is harmony. It is not enough just to have good health; we also need to feel physically in harmony emotionally and mentally. This is generally found when we achieve a state of good health and emotional and mental fulfilment. It is almost like being in love; one feels a sense of contentment and a 'oneness' between oneself and the world.

The secret of well-being is to slow down and to disconnect from the daily pressures of life. This is not a matter of switching over your concentration from one thing to another but of truly relaxing and letting go. Sometimes, the mind needs to be allowed to 'float', perhaps by listening to music or walking in the country-side. Aromatherapy can help achieve this through the inhaling of essences, such as neroli, chamomile or sandalwood, which calm the mind.

I recommend the following positive measures to maintain health:

- Take warm water with lemon first thing in the morning to help the function of the kidneys.
- Take regular exercise.
- Take walks in the fresh air, either in the park or in the countryside.
- Eat natural health-giving foods.
- Remain aware of your physical, as well as your inner, needs.
- Seek treatment for yourself when necessary.

The beauty of a woman takes on different qualities as she progresses through life. As a teenager, a woman has freshness, purity and an excitement with life which gives her vitality and a ceaseless stream of energy. She is searching for balance and equilibrium in herself. A young woman rests in herself more, and stops 'floating'. She is more tempered towards a growing maturity as she begins to appreciate her inner self. A mature woman possesses an inner understanding and a depth of feeling which she has gained from her knowledge of life. She finds a deeper way of expressing herself in relation to the world. An older woman is the sum of her life's experiences. She may retain her beauty through inner contentment and fulfilment, or display rigid features through bitterness; she may even be in danger of becoming caricatured by trying to recapture her youth.

The secret lies in not getting old, but in becoming ageless. By accepting physical changes with the advancing years a woman can radiate beauty which reflects an inner harmony in a well-shaped and well-functioning body.

Yves de Maneville

MIMI

◇ Mimi looks sporty and dynamic with her dark glasses; strong, geometric sweater; and false pony tail.

a) Divide the hair into two sections: front and back. Attach the hair piece to the crown of your head.

b) Scoop up the back section of the hair and bring the front section over the piece.

c) Finally, tie all three parts together to create your natural, long pony-tail.

a)

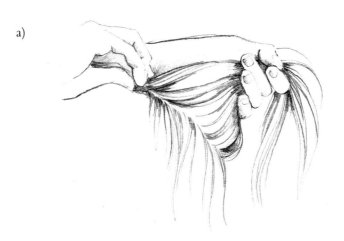

b)

c)

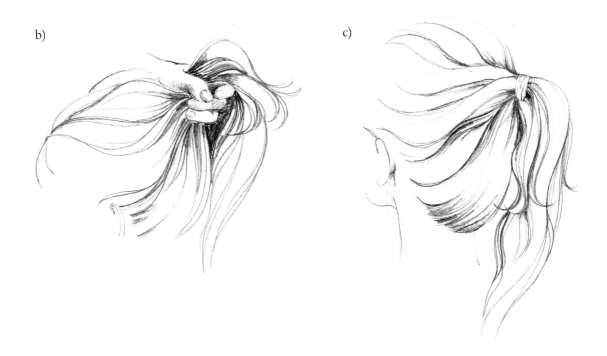

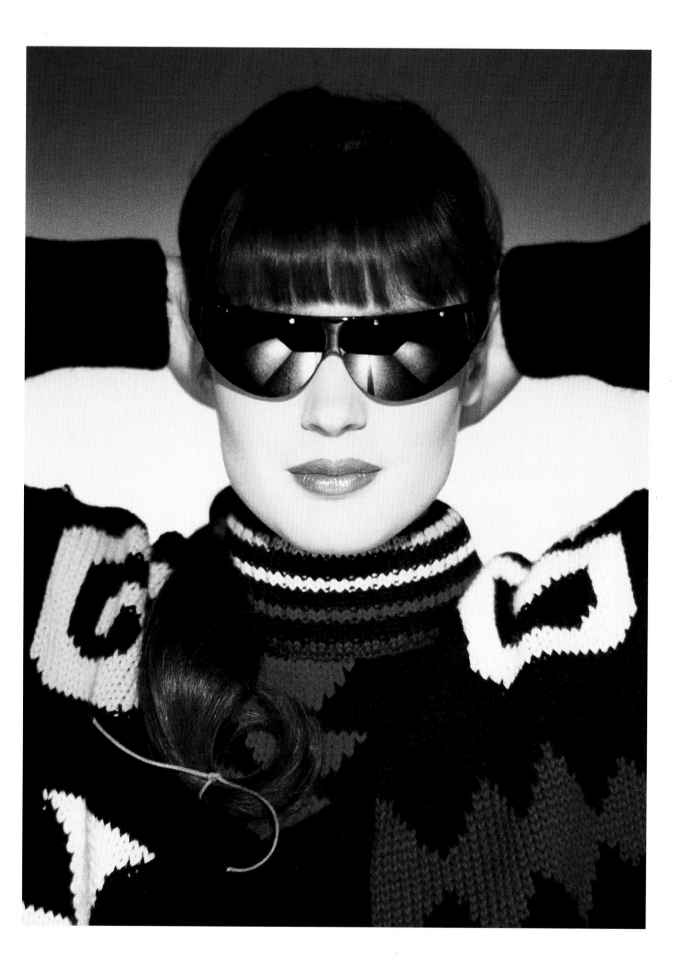

Hair for Exercise

No matter what you are doing, it is always pleasant to feel attractive and feminine. When taking exercise, whether it be jogging, aerobics, dancing or just walking the dog you will want your hair to look beautiful, be easy to manage and remain securely fastened if it is long. Simple but effective techniques are best. It is interesting to note that many of today's most successful hair accessories — such as headbands, elastics and large clips — have developed out of the need to look after hair for exercise.

When you take exercise, your body is more active and this affects the condition of your hair. For example, the sebaceous glands secrete more oil making your hair greasier. If you exercise regularly you may find that you need to wash your hair every day. If this is the case, you should only need to shampoo it once.

Divide the hair across the middle of the head. Take the front section of hair and twist in an anti-clockwise direction; knots will form naturally as you twist it. Secure the ends of the hair to the head with grips. Put a comb through the knots, as shown.

This style can be adapted for evening by placing an ornamental comb in the hair. The back could be left hanging naturally, or put up with more combs.

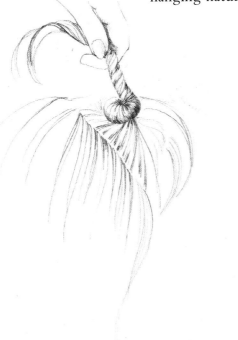

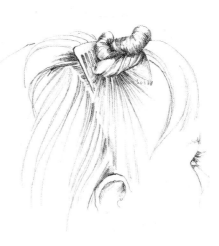

a) Tie the scarf in a knot or bow at the front and then swivel it round to the back.

b) Wrap a scarf around a pony tail and tie it in a knot.

a)

b)

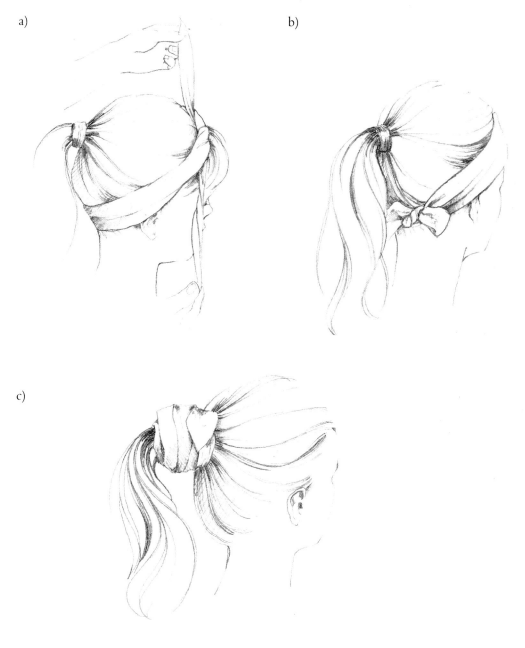

c)

c) The finished result.

a) All the hair is held in the hand, then a piece of hair is taken out from the centre of the head.

b) The hair that is taken out is wrapped around in a clockwise direction working gradually towards the head.

a)

b)

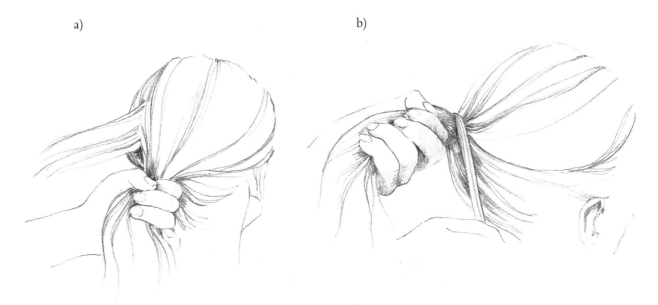

c) A hair hook is pushed under the bound section and the end is pulled through and secured.

d) The hair is safely held in place.

Hair hooks can be bought from a craft shop which sells hooks for rug making.

c)

d)

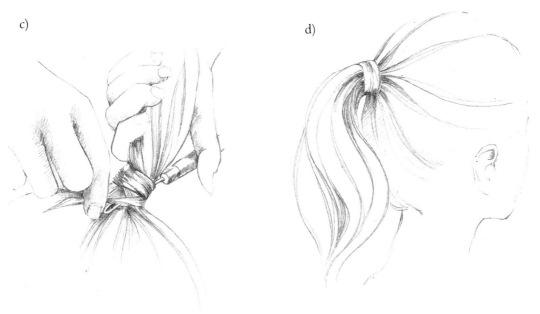

DANCE EXERCISE

My approach to movement is based on classical ballet, yoga and the Alexander technique. 'Thinking' is important — the mind and body must work as one. This brings about an 'inner awareness' and this is what I try to teach through movement, whether it be to the complete novice or to the Olympic athlete.

Every class is a new class and offers a new beginning for the mind. How one feels and what one learns during the class is something that will carry through into daily life. In a class one can work through any disturbances, upsets or emotional difficulties and feel different and more positive at the end. By doing regular exercises one is able to cope more readily with the ups and downs of everyday life. At the beginning of each class a time is spent preparing — 'centering' — the mind and body. One endeavours to find an inner quietness and to feel the balance and harmony which is naturally within our bodies, but which is often disturbed by outside tensions.

Keeping a balanced mind is essential in order to keep a healthy body. Personally, I place very little importance on diet. I listen to my body and feed it what it asks for; I think that a balanced mind encourages a balanced diet. Losing weight is just a matter of eating a little less of everything and cutting out in-between snacks. Exercise alone will not make one slimmer, but through exercise the body is toned. Muscles that are worked properly become heavier so one may actually weigh more on the scales and yet take a smaller size in clothes, because the body has become more slender.

Exercise also increases body awareness and posture; it gives the sensation of walking tall with the body carried over the legs, the head well balanced over the spine and the eyes alive and facial muscles in play. All these combine to give a feeling of vitality and happiness. Spending five minutes on a daily routine of exercise has tremendous results, more especially if done in the early part of the day so that the various muscle groups are 'woken-up' and derive day-long benefit. The exercises I prefer are those that:

● lengthen and iron out the spine
● stretch the legs, knees and thighs
● mobilise the upper body, shoulders, head and neck
● and relax the whole body.

A short sequence of exercises is a useful pick-me-up at any time of day as it relieves tension and refreshes a tired and sluggish mind.

Another contribution towards good health is an optimistic outlook on life and a sense of humour. If one is not fortunate enough to be born with these qualities they can be cultivated. A positive mind which is not dragged downwards by the possessions of life will show through the body. Fear of losing possessions and securities can manifest itself within, producing tension and tightness in joints and restricting freedom of movement. All thinking manifests itself in the body. In other words, sort out the mind and the body will sort itself out.

It is said that the beauty of a woman changes at different stages of her life. I think a lot depends on how each individual accepts and faces each challenge through-out her life. One must endeavour to learn from all experiences, at whatever age they occur, whether they be good or bad, traumatic or tragic, negative or positive. All experiences affect our emotional and mental states. It is through these experiences and how we cope with them that we become what we eventually grow into; and we keep learning until the end. My ideal is to attain an inner balance. I believe that the whole of our life is a quest to attain and maintain a balance of mental, physical, emotional and spiritual states.

Finally, relaxation and rest at the end of the day are, I think, very essential. I find that after giving so much of myself throughout the day I need a period of quietening down. Without this time I could not regain the balance of 'whole' to be able to give completely and honestly to the demands of the following day.

Margaret Kelly

JANET

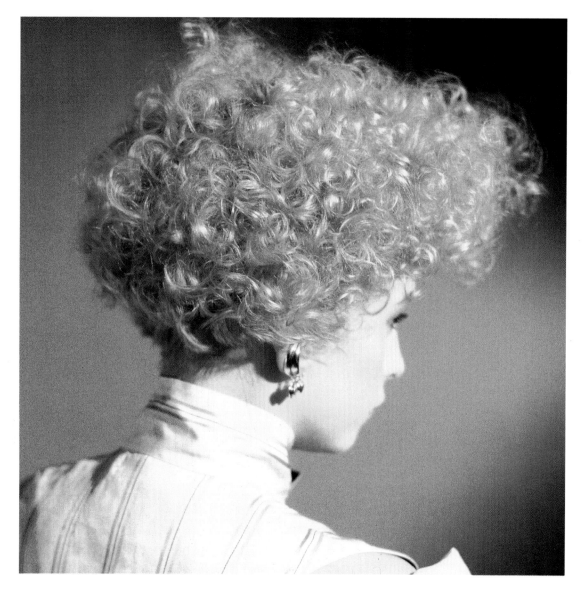

◇ Janet's naturally fine, straight hair was completely transformed by setting it dry on the smallest Molton 'permers' to create curl, volume and bubbliness.

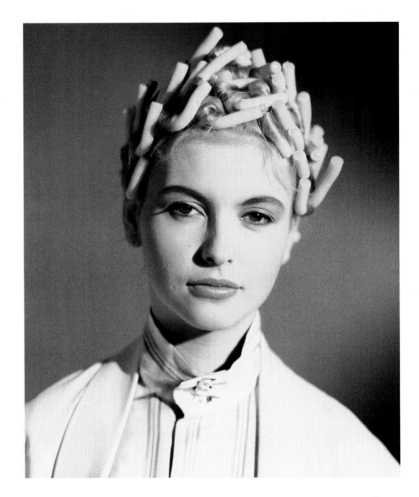

Janet shows her hair being set dry in the smallest Molton 'permers'.

○ Here is a romantic mood! The make-up describes the very pale face in gold, and soft, pink colours which tone in with the delicate, chintzy clothes. Warm-gold, pale-pink and grey shadows were used on the eyes and a pale-pink lipstick containing a gold fleck compliments the lips.

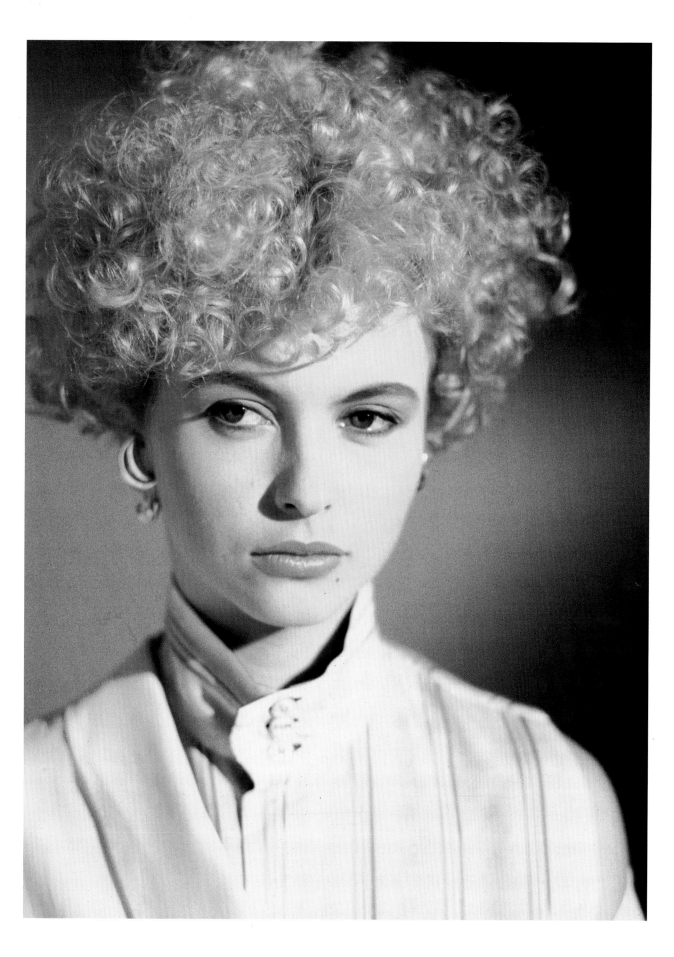

◇ Janet's hair is naturally as straight as this and it has been cut into a clean, sharp, bob.

○ Soft pinks and dusty blues emphasize the eyes and lips leaving the classic bob to speak for itself.

Fine, Straight Hair

WASHING AND DRYING

If you wash your hair daily, use very little shampoo as the hair has a tendency to dry out. The ends should be conditioned well with a light conditioner. This applies to both medium-length and short hair.

Long hair of this sort dries very quickly and so it is advisable to start the process with a towel and finish off with a blow-dryer.

CUTTING

Long hair needs to be cut rather often, at least once a month, as the ends tend to split. Medium-length hair will always look good in a bob, but it should not be over-graduated as this will make the hair look finer than it is. A short, graduated style will suit this kind of hair providing the graduation is chunky.

Often, a 'funny wave' is an indication of a 'cowslick' or a 'widow's peak', and these should be taken into account when styling the hair.

SETTING

This hair will not hold a set for more than a few hours, so perming is a good solution. Always set the hair to just the way you want it, because if you over-set it it will look droopy as the set falls out.

Medium-length hair can be set to give dramatic effects for evening (see Janet). Always use setting lotion on this kind of hair because it tends to build up static.

HIGHLIGHTING AND TINTING

This hair responds well to colouring but also knots easily. Conditioners should be used to keep it tangle-free and the hair combed with a wide-tooth comb rather than a brush.

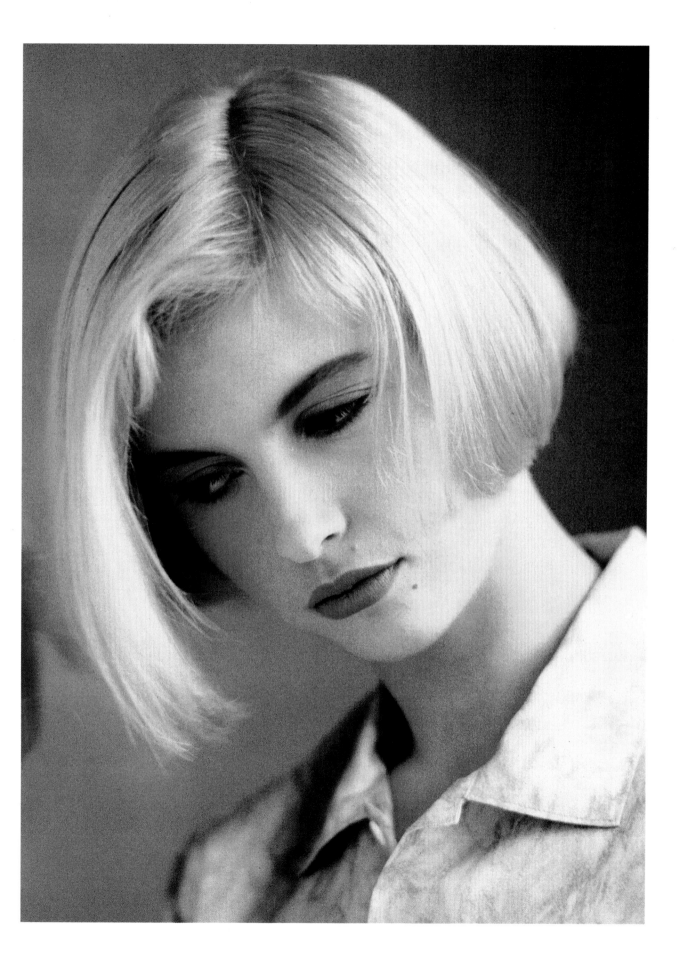

LOOKING AT HAIR

Hair is inseparable from the face and, since each face is individual, every hair-style is individual too. When I cut the hair I set out to create this link between the uniqueness of a woman's face and her hair. When I do this I take into account a woman's physical appearance: her height, her build and her posture. I look at her hair and at its colour and texture and I then study the features of her face — and look for the best ones. These might be her nose, her eyes, her mouth or her jawline. I then cut and shape the hair to enhance her best feature. This link is very subtle and it is the quality of it that makes the hair-style look 'right'. This 'rightness' is appreciated by the woman herself when she instinctively cuts a piece of hair at the top or the side of her head because she knows it is the wrong length. Although technically this is not correct, who can say that it is wrong? Many of my creative ideas for styling hair come from noticing these personal statements.

The impact of a hair-style is created by the connection between the hair and the best features of the face. To find the best feature I make a careful study of the angles of the face and I then relate these to the way I cut the hair. The best feature will influence the length of the hair-cut and the graduation. It is this subtle connection that makes the hair-style look strong and alive. As well as the best features of the face, I take into account the shape of the head. I counterbalance a round face with a narrow hair-style, a narrow face with a wider hair-style, a square face with a shape that would soften the squareness, and an oval face with a slightly squared shape. I then look at the woman's neck, her shoulders and her posture and decide on the best length for the hair to flatter those features. Hair can be likened to a shadow and the hairdresser's skill is to cut and set the hair in such a way that it affects the shape of this shadow to give height and volume, and length and width around the face.

Hair reflects something quite individual about a

woman. It is a deeply organic aspect of the body and most women would probably admit that even if they said to a hairdresser, 'I don't mind what you do to my hair,' what they really mean is, 'I don't mind what you do to my hair as long as it is right.' 'Right' means that she must feel related to the colour, the cut and the texture of her hair. It must make her feel comfortable, positive and confident about herself. 'Right' also means that the hair must be easy to look after, but versatile enough to be adapted to any kind of occasion. In short, it must relate to her lifestyle and to her mood.

When looking at a woman's lifestyle I study the clothes she is wearing, their shape, form and colour, and their relation to fashion. I take note of all these things and then we discuss her hair-style together. This gives a woman confidence and enables her to respond to any new suggestions that I might make. However, it is not possible to achieve everything on the first visit and it will take time for me to get to know her hair and to establish a confident relationship. Regular visits to the hairdresser are the only way to achieve this. From the point of view of the hair, this will ensure that it looks at its best all the time. It will also mean that I will not have to cut the hair too drastically because only a short time will have elapsed since the last visit. Becoming familiar with a woman's hair helps me to remember it better and to improve on the hair-cut each time.

There is always something new to learn, however much I may think I know. By doing a woman's hair regularly I am not restyling the hair each time, but simply reshaping it. The more I cut a woman's hair the more I appreciate it and cutting it often means that I never have to cut too much off at any one time. It is very unusual for a woman not to say, 'Don't cut my hair too short' (it is hardly ever the other way round). By this she means 'Try to remember how you cut it last time'!

Haircutting

The hair-cut is the foundation of the hair-style. Without a good cut the hair will not be able to hold the necessary volume and height for any length of time. When I cut hair I look for the form I want and even before drying it the hair should show this form. There are some types of hair I prefer to cut dry, for example, fine, blonde hair which is very difficult to see properly when it is wet. When cutting very curly hair into a fringe, I know that the hair will spring up, so I work on it dry because it is easier to see the bounce. Strong root growths in the hair can best be seen when it is dry. Sometimes, I start by cutting it dry and then check it through when it is wet. Each particular kind of hair needs to be cut differently. Sometimes it is better to cut the hair with the person standing up. I always try to cut with the shoulders exposed, as clothes will distort the way the hair falls. I look at the way a woman holds her head and if, for example, she holds it to one side, I will try to correct this before starting to cut her hair. If you do not notice this it is all too easy to cut one side shorter than the other. Then you find yourself continually trying to even up the two sides, so that in the end you have a hair-cut that is far shorter than originally planned. No cutting technique is correct for every kind of hair-style.

One technique that I use often is 'forward graduation' which tends to soften the shape of the hair-cut. If one says that the foundation of the hair-style is the hair-cut, then one could say that the foundation of the hair-cut is the technique. Although technique is not everything. The art of hair-cutting is looking. If you look as you are cutting you are more likely to notice the need for a subtle change which you could not have seen before you started. It might be a change of angle, lighter graduation, or the hair needing to be shorter. I might find the technique I am working with is limiting, so by changing the technique at this moment I am making a spontaneous decision. This is often how new techniques are developed. And all this develops from the process of looking.

There is a rhythm to haircutting which can make it very creative. By becoming sensitive to each section of hair as I work; by knowing why I am taking it and what I am doing with it; and by continually remembering why I am cutting it to the chosen length, a rhythm is created which is visible in the fluency of the finished hair-cut. If I think of the hair-cut as the foundation, and the structure as its shape and form then the result is the finished hair-style.

It can take two or three years to learn to cut hair well, and a lifetime to perfect it, so it is not really advisable for women to cut their own hair.

SETTING

Setting can be described as the way we manipulate hair. There have been great developments in this process. I have always considered it unnecessary to feel obliged to set hair wet. In the late '60s I developed a method of drying hair with the hands.

The hair-drying process is a finishing technique which lifts the hair and rolls it to give height where it is required, and flattens it where narrowness is required. The basis of the finger-drying technique relies on the fact that hair sets when it is almost dry. It is only the last few minutes that count. I will often towel dry the hair until it is damp and then start to finger dry it. If more of a set is needed I will use Molton Browners which I put in the hair when it is dry. The combination of the finger drying and the Molton Browners work together in harmony to give the desired result. Sometimes when I am finger drying the hair I will actually scrunch the hair in my hands for a few minutes before releasing it, even this movement will actually set the hair. Not every kind of hair needs to be finger dried; some hair responds better to blow drying.

First Hair-cut

Many women notice how their hair changes in texture over the years and being a part of the body, it is not surprising. Hair nearly always reflects the physical state of the person. When changes take place there is no need to worry as they are quite normal. What does not change is one's instinctive interest in one's own hair which starts at an early age.

A very small child is going to need to have its hair cut within the first few years of its life. This is a dramatic experience and can be quite frightening. It needs a lot of care and patience, and a tremendous sense of humour, so you will be looking for someone who is sympathetic and who thinks the child is more important than the hair-cut.

It is very pleasing for the child's hair to look nice, but care should be taken, at this sensitive age, to make sure that the child's well-being comes first.

Children's hair is far more important to them than we admit. This is obvious when we look at the toy industry and notice the interest in dolls and their hair. Always use good-quality products on children's hair; too strong a shampoo, for example, will dry out the scalp. Make sure that the hair is washed regularly, combed carefully, and not gripped too tightly or pulled back too fiercely. As soon as the hair has been cut once, then it should be done regularly thereafter. Resist colouring or perming a child's hair before teenage at the earliest.

During the teenage years, most young girls are eager to experiment. They are trying to find themselves, experience independence and exploring their sensuality and sexuality. They start experimenting with their life. I try neither to make a young girl look old, nor to be over dramatic in what I achieve. They want to make a statement and so do I, and achieving both is a challenge. I want to encourage their desire to explore and at the same time to direct it without limiting them.

Colour can play an important role when it comes to making a statement. There are all sorts of amazing effects which can be created and explored safely with the help of a hairdresser. It is really a question of controlling a horror story from my point of view. But I think that it is great fun to allow teenagers to try out colour and not to stifle their spirit.

A young woman begins to look for advice, whereas a teenager does not want to be told. At the same time, a young woman begins to know how she wants to look and is looking for ideas and suggestions to help her enlarge the picture of herself that she wants to project. She will choose clothes that go with this new image, and she will make decisions about this new image and keep to them for some time. Her energy is settling, and perhaps she is looking for stability in both her career and her relationships. So when I look at a young woman with a view to cutting her hair I acknowledge all this about her. She still retains much of her teenage spirit, and remembers it well. She likes to go to parties and be 'out on the town', so she is ready to have an exotic hair-style just for one evening. These moments are very creative for me and I enjoy responding to them.

A mature woman looks backward and forward at the same time. She feels her youth but she knows that she is getting older, and I need to approach her in a different way. I never try and create a 'mature' hair-style. A lot of women feel they ought to have a shorter hair cut at this age, but this is not necessarily true. I always try to be sensitive to the part in them that is youthful and, as this is usually their best feature this is what I try to enchance. A mature woman is more settled in herself and this is reflected in her lifestyle, her clothes, and her hair. When I am doing her hair I always try to encourage the positive aspects of her lifestyle. Sometimes I see a potential that is not being realized. This needs to be approached very carefully. I build up her confidence in me by going over all the positive aspects about her hair that she herself already instinctively knows. Then I will be able to suggest what I want to do and why I want to do it. This does not always work, but I think it is well worth trying. Sometimes it takes more than one visit for her to find the confidence to be willing to take this step.

An older woman does not want to be disturbed. Rather like a teenager, she does not want to be told. She has a lifelong experience of knowing her hair and does not take kindly to inexperience. She wants to have confidence in her hairdresser and to know that she is in capable hands. Her hair must be cut well, look stylish, modern and elegant. The elegance of an older woman is being able to handle situations, being able to laugh about her eccentricities, being supported by the confidence she creates around her. As a hairdresser I try to enjoy the experiences of an older woman and to enhance her positive qualities.

Every so often, for one reason or another, it is necessary to change one's hairdresser. One should never feel afraid to go to another stylist within the same salon. Sometimes a change is good, not just for the client but for the hairdresser as well. I feel that I have failed if my client comes to me and asks me to change her hair, because I feel that I should have seen this before she did. Hairdressing must be a total commitment which you renew continually by doing it. My work is as good as my last client. The focal point for me is my relationship with my client.

LOUISE

◇ Here is a soft and sensual look burnished with soft raspberry lights. The hair was finger dried and then set with Molton Browners.

Hints on Lip Colour

Both lipsticks and lip glosses are best applied with a brush. The brush distributes the lip colour evenly and when applied properly tends to last longer.

To define and correct the lip shape it is best first to line the lips with a pencil in a colour which matches your lipstick as closely as possible. If you can't find a lip pencil to match your lipstick then it is better to use a flesh-tone colour.

If you are wearing foundation, then cover the lips as well before applying your lipstick and powder lightly. If you do not wish to use foundation on your lips then apply a lip fixative, followed by a lip pencil to shape your lips; then fill in the lips with your lipstick or lip gloss. For a slightly matt finish, blot the lips with a tissue and lightly powder through the tissue.

Molton Browners

In 1976, we were trying to find a quick way of waving long hair. We tried using the traditional form of rollers, but they could not give us the right result. We experimented with pipe cleaners, and wires covered with leather, but they seemed to set the hair too tightly. We then tried covering wire with foam and fabric and suddenly found that by twisting and rolling the hair around these objects when it was dry and leaving it for

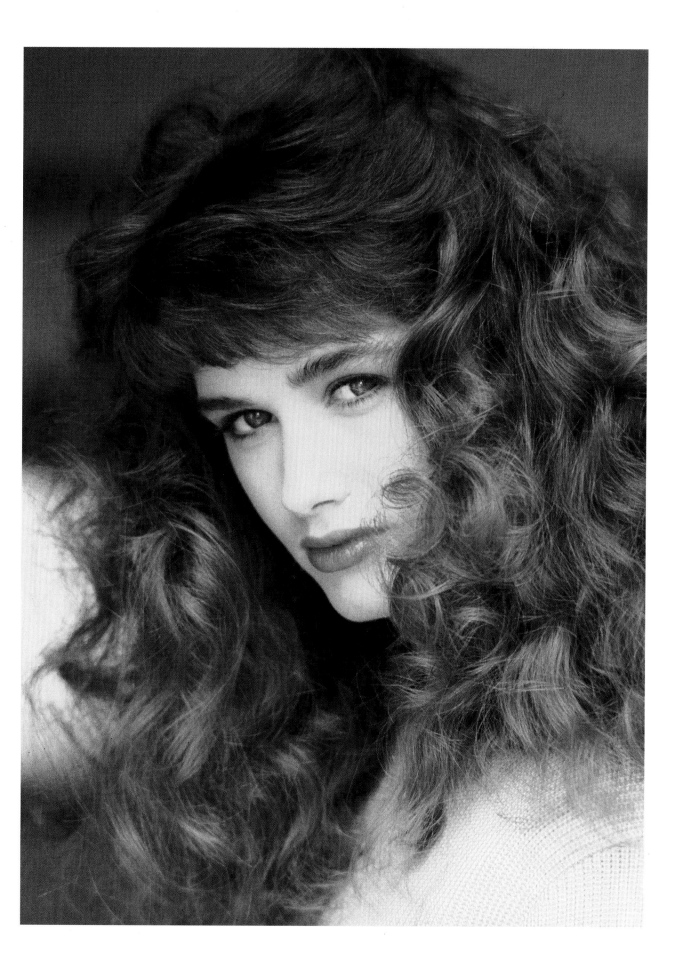

fifteen to twenty minutes, the body heat would set it. When the hair was taken out of the rollers we discovered that it had formed beautiful waves. This was the birth of the Molton Browners and the start of a method of setting hair which is now used throughout the world.

In 1980, we designed a polyethelene roller which could be used for perming hair. The principle behind it is the same as for the Molton Browner, and it now makes it possible for a woman to have her hair permed no matter how long it is. There is nothing to compare with it for flexibility and freedom. Eventually, an adaptation was made and manufactured in various different sizes for retail use; these are known as 'stylers'.

USING MOLTON BROWNERS

The hair is set in much the same way that you would set it on traditional rollers, by taking the hair in sections and winding it round the roller. There are no harsh pins and because of the long shape and soft texture of the Molton Browners, the result will be softer and more natural. To use the Molton Browner, you simply position it where you like and bend forward the two protruding ends of the roller, to secure (see opposite page).

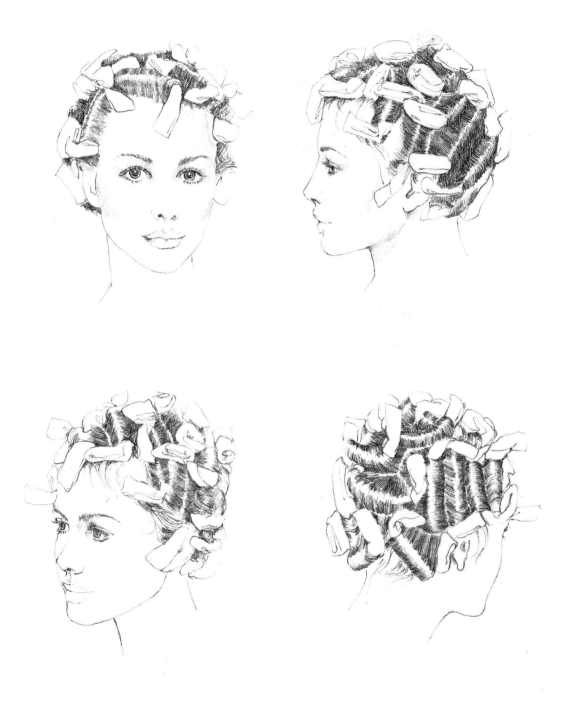

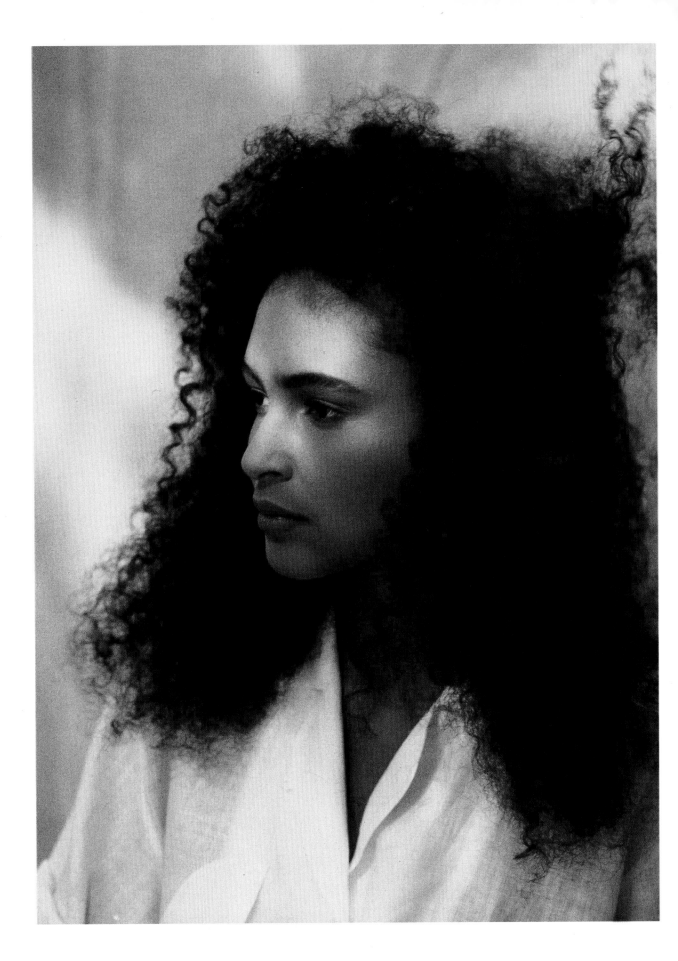

AKURA

◇ Black hair has wonderful, natural movement and does not always have to be cut short or straightened. Akura's hair was blown dry with the dryer held about a foot away from her head. It was not touched by hands, comb or brush while it was being dried. The heat of the dryer was applied under the hair to lift it and give it its own volume.

○ This is a very natural make-up based on Akura's beautiful skin tones. Using shades from the Sepia palette, the eyes were shaped and defined. An earthy-coloured blusher was brushed over the cheeks and the lips were stained with chestnut lipstick.

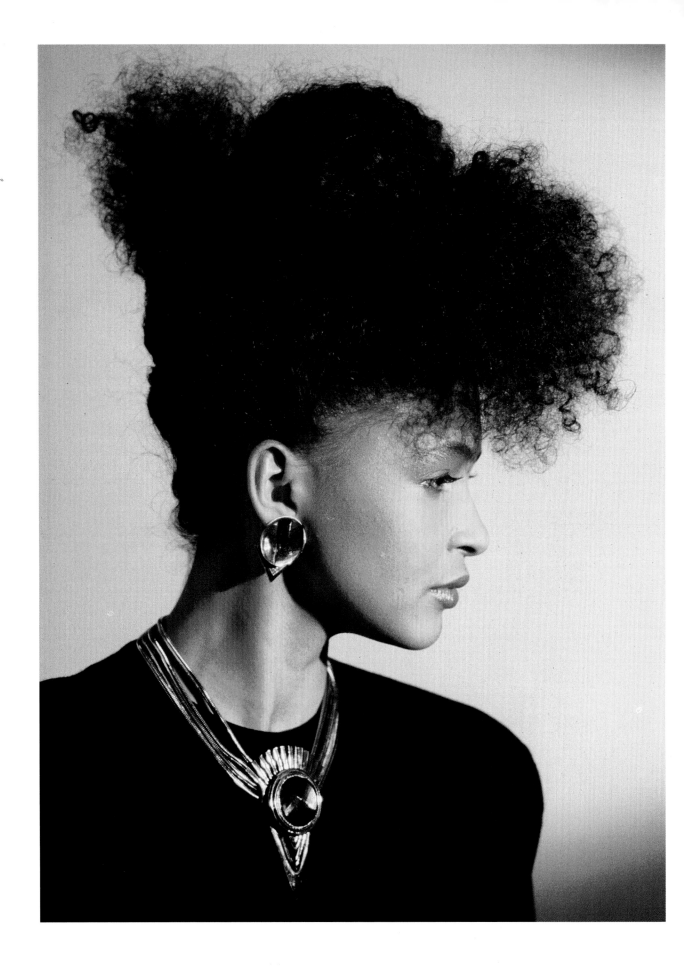

◇ Even though Akura's hair has been taken up we have allowed the individual quality of the hair to dictate its own mood.

○ Akura shows us that make-up for the evening does not have to over-exaggerate colour (although that may be what you wish to do). Here, the beauty lies in the gold, silver, pewter and other metallic shades of the eyes, cheeks and lips.

a) The back section of the hair is drawn up and folded into a pleat.

b) The remaining hair is held up …

c) and tied close to the head.

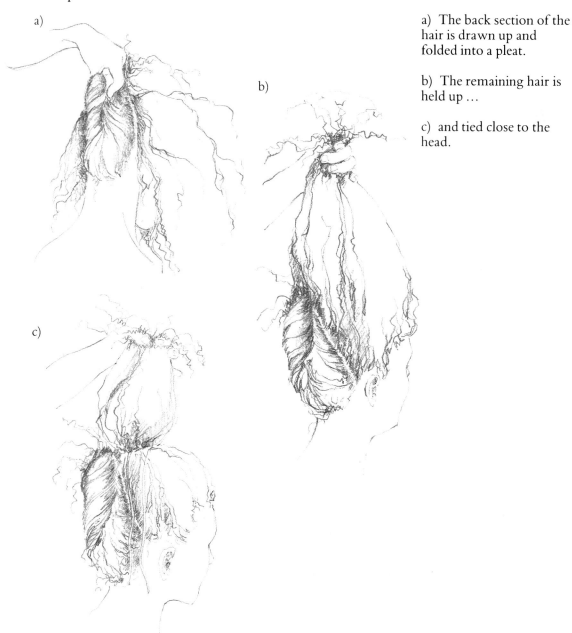

a)

b)

c)

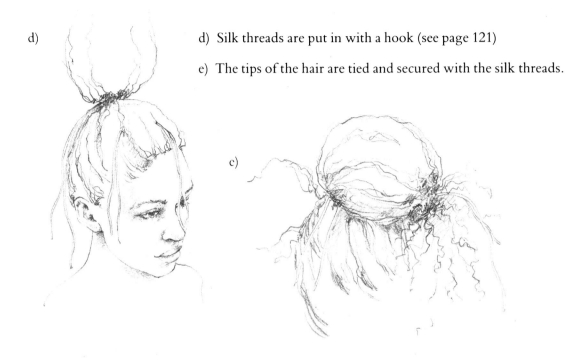

d)

d) Silk threads are put in with a hook (see page 121)

e) The tips of the hair are tied and secured with the silk threads.

e)

Coloured Skin

Black skin tends to be thicker and oilier, but the pores are finer and the texture silkier than other skins. Black skin has one great advantage over white skin which is that it ages less quickly. One of the main problems with black skin is that the colour may be uneven, which is due to the high concentration of melanin in the skin.

Coloured people should look after their skin very carefully as it tends to scar easily. As a general rule, you need to follow the same cleansing, toning, moisturizing routine as for oily or combination skin.

People with black skin can have tremendous fun with colours because they are fortunate enough to be able to wear bright, deep rich shades of eye shadow, lipstick, nail varnish and blusher. Pale colours can look good as well (see Akura page 50), but avoid those which have a chalky quality as these will make the skin look ashen. If you keep to colours that have strong pigments and little talc in them you will look stunning.

Fine, Curly, Frizzy Hair

WASHING AND DRYING

This hair needs to be washed less often because it tends to be dry. It should be conditioned well with a light conditioner after it has been shampooed. It will matt and tangle when it is washed and should be combed through with a large-tooth comb as this will not pull on the hair.

Towel drying is good for this type of hair as it will not over-dry it. The hair dries very quickly so if you do use a dryer be sure to hold it a long way from the head. In a humid climate the hair will spring up so you should use a slightly heavier conditioner which will help to counteract the tight curl that appears.

CUTTING

You should cut the hair very little if you want to wear it long, as this kind of hair always has split ends. The cut must allow for the extreme curliness of the hair and for all kinds of hairlines, both at the front and at the back. By leaving the hair longer, these features can be accommoated. Because this type of hair shrinks up, only cut it short where you want volume and height.

If the hair is short it needs to be cut in a chunky style, otherwise it can look rather fine and sparse.

SETTING

This hair takes a set very quickly and holds it well. If you wish, you can set it on large rollers which will help to take the frizz out. Remember to leave the rollers in for only a few minutes and to check them all the time, otherwise the hair will over-set.

Medium-length hair needs a minimum of setting and will hold the set for as long as the hair is clean. If you want a bouncy look which is not too curly then gently roll the hair round the brush and as you lift the brush away from the head, use the hair-dryer to dry the hair (holding the dryer 15–23 cm (6 to 9 in) away).

If the hair is short, then give it body by using setting lotion or gel.

HOMOEOPATHY

Health is a very vague and intangible thing. We rarely recognize it when we have it, but certainly miss it when we don't. For me, perfect health is a feeling of deep contentment within me, so that I am happy just to be alive and living moment by moment, despite the changes that are going on in my life. At these times my emotions are open and sensitive and not too turbulent and destructive; my mind is clear and creative; and my body is running well with no sign of 'dis-ease'.

My body is alive because it is full of energy. When we come into the world and take our first breath, energy enters and when we die this energy leaves us. Christian Samuel Hahnemann, the founder of homoeopathy, called this the 'vital force', and described one of its functions as being to maintain health in the body. This principle is the basis of all truly holistic types of medicine and although its presence is also known to conventional medicine it is rarely emphasized. It is clear that our bodies know how to take care of us, as long as they are given the right foods, exercise, air, water and contentment. How well the 'vital force' can cope with the problem is also determined by the strengths and weaknesses which are handed down to us in our father's sperm and in our mother's egg, i.e. in our genes.

Mankind has always lived in a hostile environment. In earlier days it was under attack from sabre-toothed tigers, the physical elements and infections such as tuberculosis and syphilis. Today, we are still under attack on all levels of our being. Physically, our lungs, livers, kidneys, skin and digestive organs have to deal with the greatly increased amount of potential poisons that live in our air, water and food. We also poison our metabolisms with tobacco, alcohol and drugs of various kinds. We may be weakening our resistance by exposure to electro-magnetic radiation, from such things as television and overhead pylons. We also tend to be under more stress on the nervous system because of the increased pace of life since the industrial revolution. There is good evidence, also, that we are making ourselves less able to cope with disease because our posture is faulty as a result of the furniture that we sit on. Looking at tribesmen, they usually seem to squat on the ground or sit cross legged; both these postures keep the spine straight. Instead we tend to slouch in chairs. This can lead to poor breathing, which lessens the supply of oxygen to the brain, and also probably to digestive disorders and a general lowering of the quality of impulses passed from the nerves to every tissue in the body. As far as infections go, we may have got rid of some of the big killers of the past such as smallpox, and we have contained others such as syphilis, gonorrhoea and tuberculosis, but now we seem to have AIDS and Legionnaires Disease instead. In this age of materialism, we are under pressure to go out and buy things in order to gain satisfaction rather than using meditation and deep inner contemplation to achieve this state. All these factors contribute towards an assault on our health.

It is interesting to consider how we know when our health is deteriorating. Apart from acute diseases that can happen to anybody just because of circumstance, most disease comes on over a period of time. The stages through which we pass to get to a state of breakdown of health or 'disease' show the relationship between stress and efficiency. You probably know that, to begin with, the more stimulation and pressure you are under, the better you feel. After a while, however, instead of climbing along the dotted line the graph goes over the top, as it were. This is the point of exhaustion. At this point you start to feel a slight physical lethargy and mental apathy, and you have to force yourself to get things done. You have lost your spark and it is a bit like running to keep standing still. If the causes for this are not sorted out and rectified, then you may slide further down the graph to the point where you start to develop the symptoms of an actual illness.

Once you have established that your health is deteriorating the first thing to do is to look at all the factors mentioned above and see if you can help yourself by changing your diet, getting more sleep, getting more rest and relaxation, or taking up meditation to help you cope with the problem. Above all, be kind to yourself. If you are hard on yourself this will only increase the stress and make matters worse. If you need to seek help from a doctor try to find the right person to look after your health. A good starting point is to find a doctor whom you feel has a genuine interest in your recovery and continued well-being.

Ensuring that you follow a healthy diet is a complicated issue these days. There is so much conflicting advice given about nutrition that you can hardly be blamed for being confused. The main reason for this is that no two people will thrive on exactly the same diet. Because we all have individual metabolisms, we all have individual requirements for certain items in our diet. However, having said that, there is overwhelming evidence that food eaten in the West today is not healthy. The damaging factors being too much animal fat, too much salt, and too much refined carbohydrate (sugar, white bread and flour). To make it easier to rectify this, it is worth following the twice-a-week rule. The following items should be eaten twice a week only: meat (including red and white meat), fish, eggs, cheese; other important diet rules are:

- Have no more than half a pint of milk a day.
- Use whole grain products.
- Avoid foods containing preservatives, artificial colouring and flavouring and sugar substitutes.
- Eat lots of fresh fruit and vegetables.
- Cook more fresh food.
- Buy as much food as possible that is organically grown.
- Limit fried foods to twice a week.
- Limit frozen foods to twice a week.
- Limit food cooked in microwave ovens also to twice a week.

For many people, exercise means doing aerobics or jogging, but we need to exercise all parts of ourselves — body, mind and soul. The best exercise for the soul is meditation and exposure to objects of natural beauty. You can exercise the mind by trying new ventures on a regular basis, for example going to night school, or studying some new interest at home in the evening instead of watching the television. As the oldest man in the world (who died recently in Japan) showed us, life which is hard with lots of physical exercise, a simple diet and a healthy sex life does wonders for us. Sex is certainly one of the things that you do not have to restrict to twice a week.

Each stage in a woman's life brings new challenges. In the adolescent years, when the body is still developing, it is usually free from ill-health. The main problems which detract from your beauty are likely to be the turmoil of working out your sexuality and the shyness, embarass-ment, and insecurity that accompany that process. This is often heightened by unhappy experiences in romance, which can leave you feeling broken-hearted and dis-traught. If you feel like this try to treat the whole thing as a learning process rather than as the end of the world; and try to take notice of other people rather than dwelling on yourself.

As you get into your twenties and thirties you may have a job or career, you may get married and you may become pregnant. Each situation will bring its own stresses and new problems to be dealt with. Pregnancy is as turbulent in its effect as puberty, and it may be difficult to reconcile yourself with the changes in the body that you see looking at you from the mirror. This is not a permanent state of affairs, however, and with careful diet and exercise you can recover your former glory. Try to accept things as they are.

As you reach the menopause and beyond, you will find that your metabolism tends to slow down, your skin begins to lose its elasticity, and wrinkles start to appear. This should not be a cause for deep concern since the part of you which is suffering from the changes is not the deepest part of you, which is still at peace and inside you. It is difficult sometimes to keep this perspective and you will have to work harder at nutrition and exercise in order to keep yourself in shape. Try and grow old with dignity, however. If you are at peace within yourself that quality will shine out through your eyes and make you an attractive woman.

Dr Lockie, M.F. Hom., M.R.C.G.P.

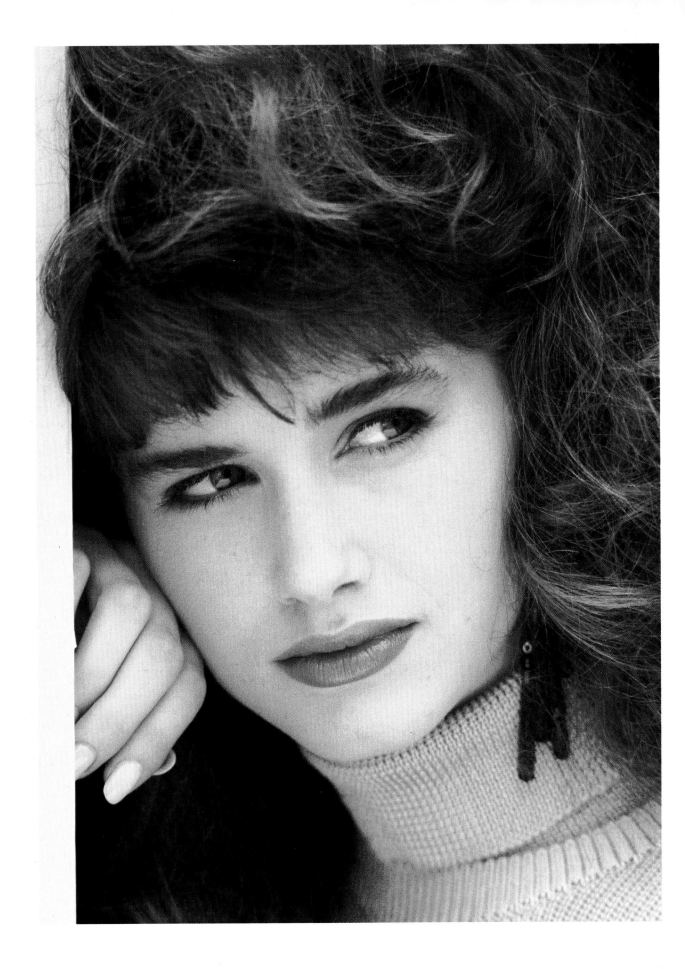

LOUISE

◇ This warm, sensual look is enhanced by the hair's soft raspberry·lights.

○ This is a day-time make-up.

Eyes A soft, lilac shade was brushed all over the eye, then a fresh, mint-green colour, slightly stronger than that of her sweater, was added in a line across the top of the eyelid. Following this, a paler, mint-green shadow was brushed over the lid to soften it, removing any trace of a hard line. Green mascara was used on the top lashes to accentuate the green liner.

Blusher A very soft, lavender-pink blusher was skimmed over the cheeks.

Lips Raspberry-pink lipstick was applied, and then blotted to remove the shine.

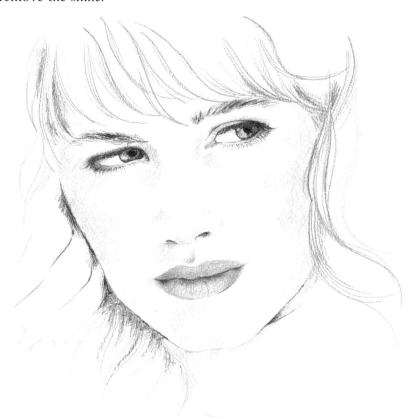

Natural Cosmetics

The term natural cosmetics is often used as a marketing ploy to create an image of wholesome products. Compltly natural products are not only aesthetically unpleasant but they do not survive even the shortest time on the shelf. Where water is present, preservatives are essential to prevent deterioration. Although many natural plant oils have benefical properties they are generally not used alone, as they are often greasy and can cause irritation if undiluted. Natural colours are available and some are used by the cosmetic industry but many fade quickly in sunlight, and colour cosmetics would be very dowdy if inorganic pigments were omitted.

Unfortunately, the chemical industry has a bad reputation, and we are wary of using chemicals (often through fear of the unknown). However, many naturally occurring materials, for example salt, and even the human body, are in fact chemicals.

Science has a great deal to offer. Skin care, particularly, has benefited from advances made in research during the past few years. On the other hand, plant extracts have been used effectively by man for centuries, and although we may not always know why they work, they undoubtedly do. To disregard all that is past or all that science can offer, would be folly. The ideal solution is to achieve a balance by extracting the best from both fields.

ANIMAL EXTRACTS AND TESTING METHODS

There is now considerable public awareness about the welfare of animals. Molton Brown have never used animal extracts, by which we mean slaughtered raw material such as animal placenta or collagen. However, we allow the use of by-products which do not harm the animal, such as honey and beeswax.

It is a Molton Brown policy *not* to use animals for testing either ingredients or finished products. We believe that the tests carried out on animals (such as Driaze testing) are in many cases not even related to the in-use 'test' carried out by consumers. Dermatological testing gives a much truer indication of the irritancy factor of a product and therefore our products are independently tested on human candidates by a British university . This is more expensive than animal testing, as human volunteers have to be paid. However, as well as being more humane, it also gives a more accurate result. Even the S.P.F. (Sun Protection Factor) testing of our sun care lotion was carried out this way.

PATTERNS OF IRRITANCY

Although known irritants are avoided, it is impossible to formulate a cosmetic product that no one will react to. In the same way that some people cannot eat certain foods, some individuals react adversely to certain cosmetics. Fragrances alone are notorious for causing irritancy in some people and although we have left our skin care or colour cosmetics without fragrance, what would a foam bath or body lotion be like without a fragrance? Certainly less luxurious!

Since cosmetics, by their very nature, are often applied to sensitive areas, people who are prone to irritancy should try any new product on the inside of the wrist or neck for twenty-four hours. Normally, any reaction will show up in this time.

COLOUR

Molton Brown cosmetics are designed to enhance a woman's beauty, rather than to make her look as if she is wearing a painted mask.

The products are formulated so that they are light in texture and a pleasure to wear. The tinted moisturizers feel completely natural; and the face powders, blushers and eye shadows are hand-sifted to make them ultra-light and soft to apply. Lipsticks are glossy and moisturizing and the natural mascara deepens and darkens the lashes evenly. When a woman applies make-up she should not only look more attractive but still look herself. The ultimate compliment should be, 'You look lovely today!' and not simply, 'Your make-up is lovely!'

RICHENDA

◇ Here, the hair has been put up into a French pleat, but the natural movement in the front has been kept in order to give volume and height. In a subtle way it gives the impression of a short hair cut.

○ This is a day-time, city make up. The monochromatic look is created by using eye shadows, lip colours, and cheek colours from a single range. In this case, the tones are warm and earthy and pick up the colours in the hair and skin. (You can also create a monochromatic look with coral hues and dusty pinks.)

Eyes A fawn–coloured eye shadow was brushed over the entire eye, followed by a soft-brown colour on the upper eyelid. Then a darker brown shadow was smudged along the base of the upper lashes and carried on under the lower lashes. The mascara was brown.

Cheeks A flesh-tone blusher was used to add shape rather than stark colouring.

Lips Chestnut lipstick was applied with a brush, blotted with a tissue, then powdered over the top to give a soft, matt effect.

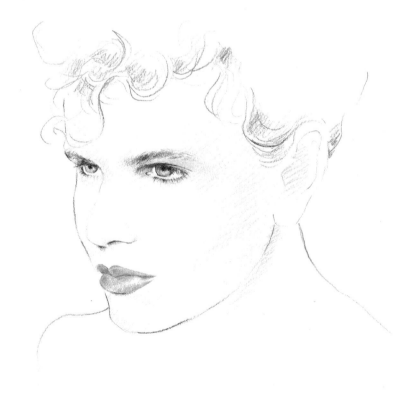

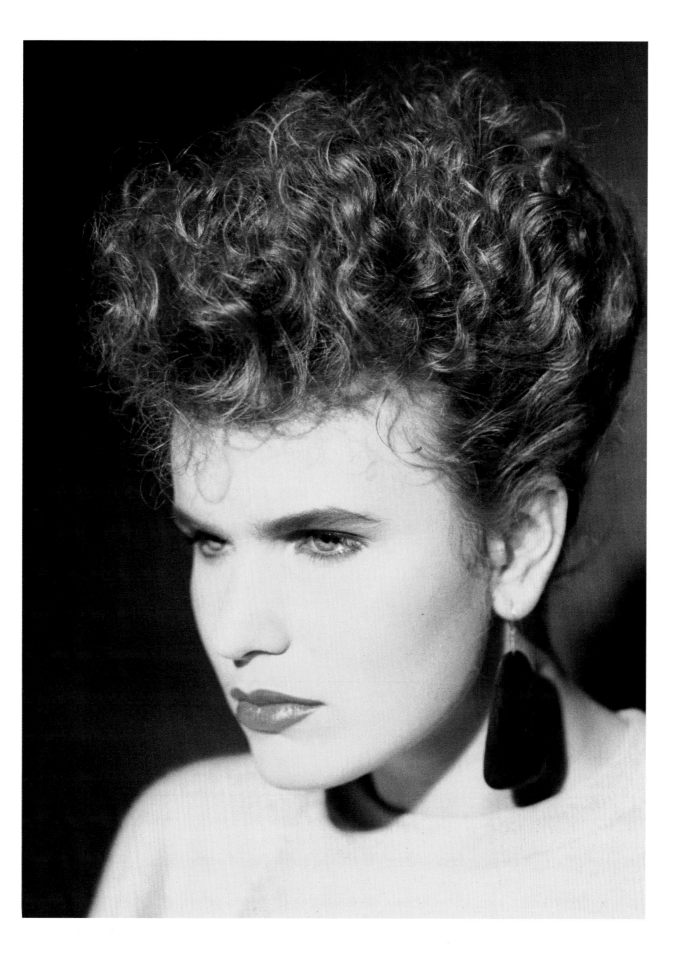

INSPIRATION FOR COLOUR

People often ask me how I arrive at the colours I have chosen. There is no single answer to this question as a great many different elements contribute to my final choice. I think possibly I am a frustrated artist! But from as far back as I can remember I have felt passionate about colours and textures. As a child, my bedroom was crammed full of sea shells, pebbles and rocks that I had fallen in love with on the beach because of their wonderful colours and designs. It was the same with leaves and flowers. The books in the house would be full of precious flowers being pressed as I tried to preserve the life of a leaf, a petal or a blade of grass. I am sure that I am not the only one who finds that all these elements provide a deep sense of satisfaction and real joy. I have always been surrounded by the world of fashion and I remember being fascinated by samples of odds and ends of fabric which were brought home to me as a young child. The education I received from my parents and their surroundings helped to develop in me an instinctive love and appreciation of beautiful fabrics and interesting textures.

The combination of all these things have provided me with an invaluable background to working with colour and texture. When I launched into the world of make-up I found I had a wealth of material inside me that I could call upon and express creatively.

The colours we choose are often influenced by fashion, but at the same time I have to make sure that a colour is wearable when it is interpreted into make-up. It is very important that the shade we use complements and enhances the face, and is not simply a fashion statement totally unrelated to the wearer. Perhaps this is why I found that my favourite shades have always been inspired by nature or from natural objects in the environment.

To formulate the colours needed I work by the side of our cosmetic chemist who, to my mind, is the equivalent of a cordon bleu chef. Together we cook up the new season's shades. To make powder eye shadows and blushers, we work with very fine talc that has been ground three times and then been sifted. While we are working, we have in front of us the object which inspires us—this might be a pebble or a flower. We have a large selection of raw pigment as well as base iridescent shades and it is the subtle blending of these essential ingredients that will eventually give us the correct shade, depth and texture.

For lipsticks, a different process is required. There are far fewer pigments to choose from. In fact, every single lipstick shade you find is created from five or six base pigments. These pigments are blended with waxes, and we include beeswax. To add shimmer to a lipstick we will add the same iridescent powder that goes into the eye shadow.

Our most popular eye shadows followed a soft-pink and soft-yellow theme and were inspired by some sea shells that I found on the beaches of Long Island. Another success was a range of purple and grey eye shadows inspired by the tiny pebbles discovered on a deserted Pembrokeshire beach. The close study of red and pink fuschias has given us some of our richest and brightest lipsticks, whereas rose petals, honeysuckle, leaves and even certain barks have been the source of inspiration for some of our neutral skin tone shades. From our environment we created a grey eye shadow from the deep grey of slate roof tops. Our lipstick called London Brick was literally inspired by the famous red brick. One of our unusual colour combinations grew out of efforts to achieve the shades of a bruise. We created a yellow-beige, a smudgy-purple and soft-navy. These shades are so much a part of the natural skin tones found around the eye area that, when applied as eye shadows, they create the illusion of wearing no make-up at all. Yet the eyes appear beautifully shaped and defined.

Now, Molton Brown has a library with hundreds of colours. Each season when we are working on the new colour range, I always imagine that the shade must already exist in our library. But in fact, the particular subtlety I am searching for is never quite present in the old shades. So each new season means a new beginning.

Caroline Collis

APPLYING MAKE-UP

Make-up is a wonderful and exciting way of enhancing your features and it is perfectly possible to achieve a natural look as well as a high fashion look. The natural look is not a face devoid of make-up but one that simply does not look 'made-up'. You can be wearing foundation, eye shadows, blushers, lipstick and mascara and still look wonderfully 'natural'. So, while most of us need to wear make-up, it is the way in which we apply it, the subtlety of the tones we use, and how we harmonize it that will make all the difference.

FOUNDATION AND TINTED MOISTURIZERS

Foundation and tinted moisturizers are designed to even out your skin colour. The important difference between them is that a foundation is heavier than a tinted moisturizer. When choosing either, try to match your skin colour as closely as possible, because if you don't you will look unnatural right from the start.

A tinted moisturizer is exactly what it says, a moisturizing cream with a touch of colour pigment added. Because it is so light, it is ideal for young skin and for skin which is virtually blemish-free. It will even out and enliven your natural skin tone and you should neither look nor feel as if you are wearing make-up. It is ideal for use in the summer to give your skin a warm glow.

Foundation is a denser product because it contains talc or titanium. It should go on smoothly and will cover blemishes and even out your skin tone to give you a flawless base. It can be used all over the face but if you are not careful, or if the shade is not quite right, it can look obvious and heavy. So it is best restricted to the areas where it is needed, such as under the eyes or where there is a blemish. You can apply foundation with your finger-tips or, better still, with a damp latex sponge.

POWDERS

There are many different kinds of powders available designed to suit all the different skin types. The shades vary from pale to dark and you can even find pastel-colour shades. However, the easiest to use and the most popular is a translucent powder which does not alter the skin tone at all. Applied over a base or on its own, a translucent powder helps blushers and eye shadows to go on more smoothly and also helps to take the shine off the face. The powder should be used very lightly, and the main areas to apply it are on the eyelids, cheeks, nose and chin.

EYES

The main reason for making up your eyes is to define and compliment the shape. You can use bright colours or natural shades. Eye shadow is your key accessory in all make-up because it offers the widest range of colours and is, therefore, very versatile.

Eye shadow comes in a variety of shades and forms: cream, powder and iridescent. Powders are the easiest to apply as they give you more control and a softer effect than the cream. A cream tends to get caught in the creases of your eye. Iridescents can seem messy and uncontrollable at first but, with a little practice, they can add a new shimmer which is perfect for use in the evening.

BLUSHER

Blusher is used primarily to add colour to your face and to emphasize the structure of your cheekbones. The danger here is the tendency to use too strong a colour and to be heavy-handed. It is important to blend your blusher so that you cannot see where it begins or ends.

The powder form of blusher is the most popular and the easiest to use. However, the other two have their uses: the gel stays on for longer, but is difficult to apply; and the cream is good for drier skin but gets absorbed and fades very quickly.

LIP COLOUR

Lip colour adds the finishing touch to your make-up. It also prevents your lips from drying out. Lip colours come in a wide array of shades and in two basic forms — lipstick and lip gloss. Lip colours look different on each person, so always test them before you buy them. Experiment with colours and finishes — matt, shiny, frosted or opaque — until you find one that suits each of your moods. Lipstick consists primarily of oil, beeswax and pigment. A lip gloss contains more oil than a lipstick and looks lovely on young people because it is light and sheer. It can give a natural look to the lips when blotted and is particularly pretty in summer.

BASIC MAKE-UP SEQUENCE

a) Check eyebrows for stray hairs and then shape. The shape of the eyebrows should compliment your face.

b) *Concealer* Lighten dark areas under the eyes and cover spots or blemishes with a concealer that is slightly lighter than your skin tone.

a)

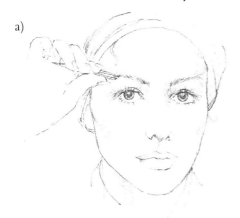

b)

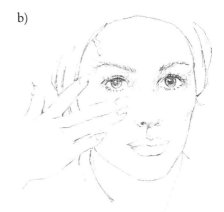

c)

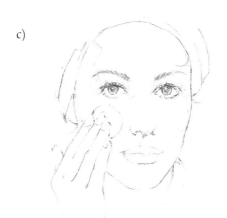

c) *Foundation or Tinted Moisturizer* Use a foundation or tinted moisturizer which matches your skin tone. Blend evenly with a damp sponge or fingertips. Use the palm of your hand as a palette to make the consistency more manageable; this warms the liquid so that it goes on smoothly. You can use tinted moisturizer all over the face. Foundations can be used either as a concealer on the areas where you feel it is necessary, or all over the face.

d) *Powder* Powder your face lightly with translucent powder using a puff or a large brush.

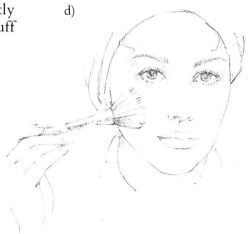

e) Brush and fill in the eyebrows using either a pencil or else powder eye shadow applied with a brush. Use light feathery strokes and if you are using a pencil, make sure it is sharp.

f) *Eye shadow* Apply light shadow all over the eyes, from the lashes to the brow, to act as a base. This makes colour blending easier for the steps that follow.

e)

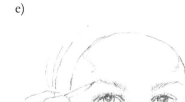

f)

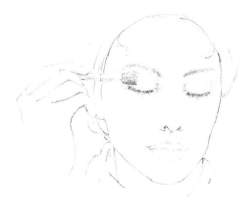

g) Add other colours to the eyes as you wish using a combination of dark shadows, bright colour or eyeliner that appeals to you.

h) *Eye pencil* To add emphasis, put the eye pencil on the outer corners of the eye; and for a softer effect, smudge with a brush or cotton bud.

g)   h)

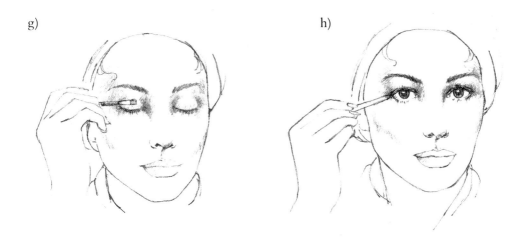

i) *Mascara* Apply mascara to top lashes only. Then continue with the rest of your make-up going back to do the lower lashes at the end. This allows the mascara to dry on the top lashes and eliminates spotting and smudging.

j) *Blusher* Powder blusher is the quickest and easiest to use. Taking into account the shape of your own face, apply blusher to the cheek bone, blending both above and below so that there is no hard stripe.

i)   j)

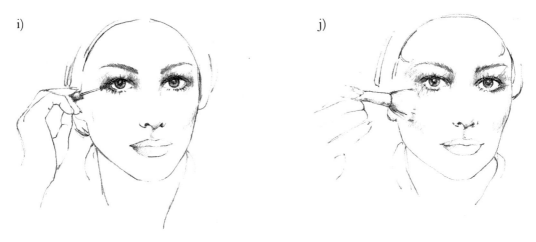

k) *Lips* Outline lips with a lip pencil to even up, or improve the shape of the lips. This defines the lips and helps prevent lipstick or gloss from bleeding.

l) Apply lipstick or lip gloss with a lip brush as this gives better definition. If a matt effect is desired, blot with a tissue and powder lightly.

k)

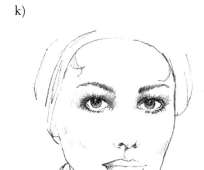

l)

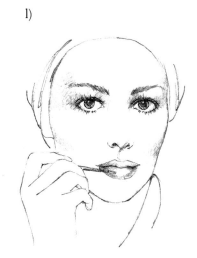

LIPS

Thin lips If your lips are thin, outline them just outside the natural lip line with a flesh-toned pencil, or a pencil that matches your lipstick. If you over exaggerate the shape of your lips you will draw unwelcome attention to them! Fill in with the lip colour of your choice

Too full lips If your lips are too full, line them just inside your natural lip shape with a flesh-toned pencil, or a pencil that matches your lipstick. Matt lip colours tend to make your lips appear smaller, so here is a hint: to make lipstick look matt, separate a tissue so that you have a very thin sheet, place this over your mouth and apply powder over it. Now remove the tissue and lightly brush off any excess powder. This will give you a perfect matt finish.

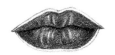

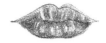

Uneven lips If your lips are uneven, you can correct the imbalance using a flesh-toned pencil, or a pencil that matches your lipstick. A good way to check that both sides are even is to blot them, with your mouth closed, on a tissue.

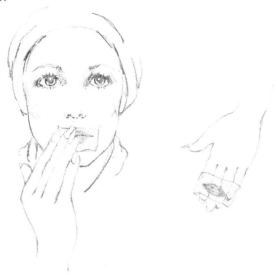

EYES

There are no fixed rules about making up your eyes, but here are some general guidelines for the six basic eye shapes. Many people will find that they have a combination of more than one of the basic shapes: for example, close-set eyes may also be droopy, and wide-set eyes may also be deep-set.

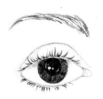 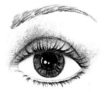

Protruding eyes look as if they extend too far out of the eye sockets. To correct this, use dark, smoky, matt colours which absorb the light on eyelids and browbone. Avoid frosted shadows and light shadows on their own. When you use dark or smoky shadow, cover the eyelid and blend it into the crease and brow area; continue applying it lightly, just two-thirds of the way along the lower lashes. Line the outer half of the upper and lower lashes with a dark shadow.

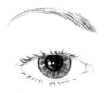

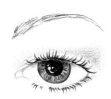

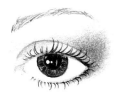

Deep set eyes are set deep into the eye sockets with the browbone appearing to dominate. To correct this, use light-reflecting colours such as bright, iridescent, light shadows on the lid. Use a thin line of colour along the base of the lashes and on the lid. Make the browbone recede by using non-shimmery shadows. Never use dark eye liner or pencil on the lid as this will cause the eye to appear even deeper set. If you do use eye liner on the outer corner of the eye, smudge it to soften the effect.

Small eyes are those which seem small relative to the shape of the face. To correct this use light shadow on the lid, and blend a darker shade on the outer half of the eye, taking it up into the browbone and out past the actual eye area. Blend the shadow part of the way along the lower lashes to make them look thicker. Curl the eyelashes.

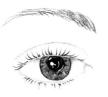

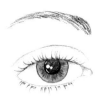

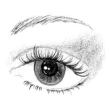

Wide-set eyes are the opposite of close-set eyes. There is more than enough, or too much, space between the eyes and the bridge of the nose. To correct this, shade in a dark eye shadow between the eyes and the bridge of the nose. You can bring the eyebrows slightly closer towards the middle by filling them in with pencil or eye shadow.

Droopy eyes slope downwards. To correct this, be sure to use upward motions when applying eye shadow. Stop the eye liner just before you reach the end of the top lashes. Apply shadow under the lower lashes and when you come to the corner, blend it upwards. A good tip is to use foundation or concealer on the outer corners before applying any eye make-up.

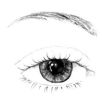

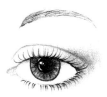

Close-set eyes appear to be very close together with little space between the eyes and the bridge of the nose. To correct this, use light, highlighting colours on the eyes near the bridge of the nose. Avoid using dark eye liners in the inner corners of the eye. Pluck the eyebrows away from the nose.

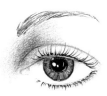

RICHENDA

◇ This long, dark blonde hair is naturally curly and was blown dry with the dryer held a foot away from the hair. It is very important not to touch this type of hair while it is being dried. By drying the hair in this way the curls remain intact and the hair falls naturally.

○ This is a day-time make-up in warm and earthy, brown, copper and gold tones which complement the skin and the warmth of Richenda's hair.

Colouring and Perming

Both colouring and perming create a dramatic change to your hair and to the way you look. Before taking the decision to have either of these treatments, there are a number of influential factors to take into consideration. In the long run, these will prove more important than whether a particular colour or perm is in fashion.

Whether going to a salon or doing your own hair at home always ask yourself the following questions:

- Is your natural skin-tone and eye colouring going to match and complement your chosen colour?
- Is your usual make-up going to complement, or clash with, your chosen hair colour?
- Will your lifestyle, job and clothes suit your prospective hair colour or style?
- If you are having a perm do you know how to make it look its best?
- Will you need to blow dry your hair to achieve your desired result? If so, do you have time to blow dry your hair?
- Do you fully understand the importance of looking after the condition of your coloured or permed hair?

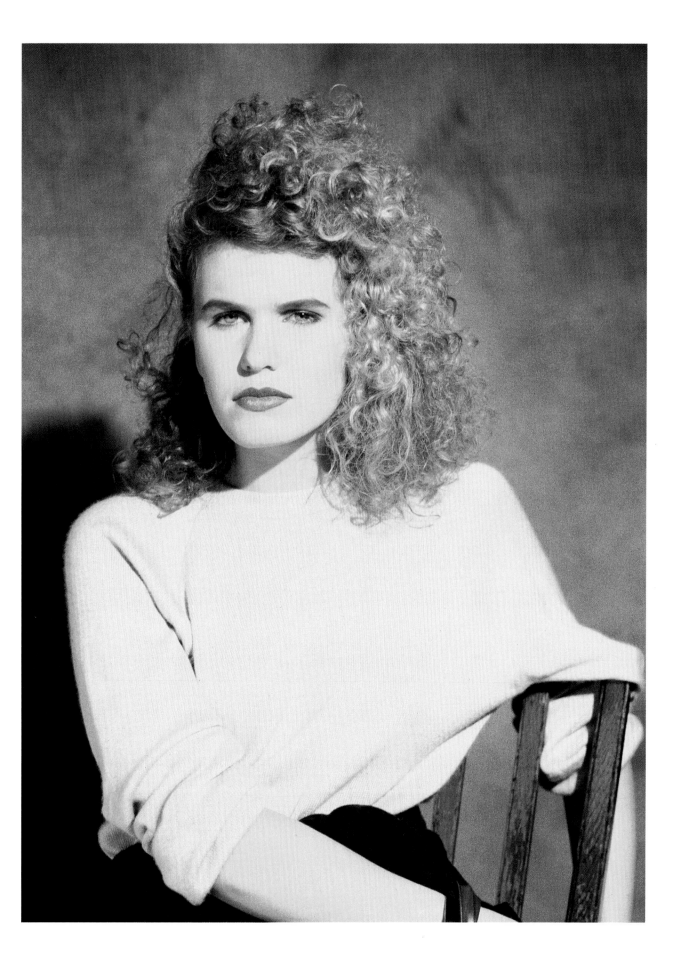

It is important to resolve all of these potential problems at the initial consultation. It is surprising how few people think practically when choosing a new look. If you are thinking of a major change to your hair, discuss it with your hairdresser, as it is always beneficial to exchange ideas.

COLOURING

If you buy a product from the chemist, with the intention of colouring your own hair, make sure that you read the contents and instructions first. As a rough guideline, whenever there are two bottles which need to be mixed together this will be a tint; if only one bottle is needed, this will be a rinse.

Tints are a form of permanent colour that only work with the addition of peroxide or a similar chemical activator. A tint enters through the outer layer, or cuticle, of your hair and goes into the cortex where it alters and combines with the natural colour pigment. A tint can totally change the natural colour of your hair or cover grey hair up to a hundred per cent, depending on the colour chosen. However, there will be a definite re-growth that will need touching up every four to six weeks.

Rinses cover a slightly wider spectrum, ranging from herbal rinses and temporary colours to semi-permanent colours. Natural and herbal hair rinses will not affect the basic colour of your hair but will enhance the natural pigments and add gloss. Vinegar and beer rinses may be used on dark or red hair, whereas lemon or chamomile are suitable for fair hair. Temporary rinses, such as coloured setting lotions and water rinses, give a coloured coating to the outside cuticle layer of the hair and do not penetrate any further unless the hair is very porous. They will wash out with the next shampoo, but they are good for adding subtle colour tones to the hair for a special occasion or for brightening up fading highlights.

Semi-permanent rinses can cover grey hair up to sixty to seventy per cent. They can give depth and warmth or be used to bring out natural highlights. They contain neither peroxide nor ammonia and cannot, therefore, lift the natural pigment. These rinses are, perhaps, the best introduction to colour change as they gradually fade out with each wash and last about four to six weeks, leaving little or no regrowth line.

Fun colours are products that are harmless and fun to use — spray colours being the most common. These come off with your next shampoo unless your hair is particularly porous, in which case it may take a few shampoos to remove them. Glitter dust is good for the evening and can either be sprayed on or applied to individual areas. You can even use eye shadow glitter by mixing it with a little hair gel and stroking it on with an eyebrow brush.

Choosing colour, whether it is to be permanent or temporary, should be undertaken with care. Colour descriptions on products sold in a chemist's can be confusing. In general, try to choose a colour one or two shades lighter than you actually want because colours are usually darker than you anticipate. When colouring fair or grey hair, beware of anything that says 'warmth' as this usually means 'red'. If you want to add warmer tones to your hair, this can be done by mixing a base colour with a tonal, e.g. mid-brown and mid-warm-brown will give you a mid-brown with chestnut overtones.

Herbal rinses, semi-permanent rinses, and some tints are the only home treatments I would recommend you attempt yourself. Anything more adventurous, such as bleaching, streaking or perming should always be carried out by a professional. In a salon, it may be difficult for the client to understand professional terminology and as a result, she may end up with something she does not want. Here is a guide to understanding your hairdresser:

Streaking Your hairdresser will probably refer to 'high-lighting' or 'lowlighting' rather than streaking. Technically, highlights are bleached strands of hair (these give a much lighter ivory tone) and are really only suitable for hair which is in the colour range of light brown up to naturally fair. Bleached streaks on any hair colour darker than this will give the impression of being prematurely grey. Lowlights are tinted strands of hair and can, therefore, range in colour from blue-black to red to golden blonde, depending upon your own original base colour and shade of tint chosen. I like to use at least two or three different colours to maintain as natural a result as possible (hair naturally has at least four or five different colours running through it).

Streaks can be achieved by several different methods. The foil method makes it possible to work much closer to the root, to emphasize a particular hairstyle, to use as many colours as required, to avoid colour build-up and breakage on the ends and to keep control over the work. Foil streaking is a more time-consuming and costly method, but the results are well worth it.

Bleaching Very few salons offer a bleaching service these days. This is mainly due to damage caused to the hair by whole-head bleaches and also because of the improvement in professional tinting products which now make it possible to produce high degrees of lift. Bleaches work by totally destroying the natural colour pigments in the hair. In doing this, they also damage some of the main hair structure. This can often result in porous, dry, and often broken hair.

Perming In the last few years the quality of perms and perming products have improved tremendously and they can now be used to create a wide variety of looks, from natural body and texture to wild corkscrew curls. Whatever look you are aiming to achieve a perm is best done professionally as any damage caused to the structure of the hair cannot be repaired. A perm works by breaking down the links in the hair that keep it straight and reforming them around a curler to give a long-lasting movement. This chemical process requires careful application and timing. Most problems encountered with perms today are caused by the after-care treatment at home. So here are some hints on how to look after your perm:
● To obtain the best results from a 'wash and leave' perm, shampoo every day with a mild shampoo, condition the hair, and comb through with the conditioner on. Rinse thoroughly and re-apply a little conditioner to the ends of hair and leave in. Comb through and towel dry hair, then scrunch up with hands to obtain maximum bounce and curl. Mousse or gel can be used to give curls a more individual look or hair can be scrunched with hands and a hairdryer to give a wilder look.

● If you prefer to set your hair or if you use any form of heat to dry it then it is important to have periodic treatments to maintain the condition. If you use heated rollers then be careful with them; cut off the spikes (because they tear your hair), and cover the rollers with very thin foam. Always aim to avoid using too much heat on the hair, and try not to pull it too much when drying it. Both of these will adversely affect the condition and look of your perm.

● Never brush the hair after it has been permed and if you comb it, do so very gently. Always leave at least forty-eight hours before shampooing the hair to avoid the perm dropping. (It takes forty-eight hours for the protein in the hair to 'harden' after a perm.)

● When you are on holiday, whether looking after permed or coloured hair, always be thorough with both shampooing and conditioning so that you remove all traces of sand or salt. If you are swimming in a highly chlorinated pool, always ensure that your hair is thoroughly rinsed afterwards as some hair colours can be adversely affected by chlorine. Finally, always try to use a protector or sun filter on your hair to deflect the sun's rays.

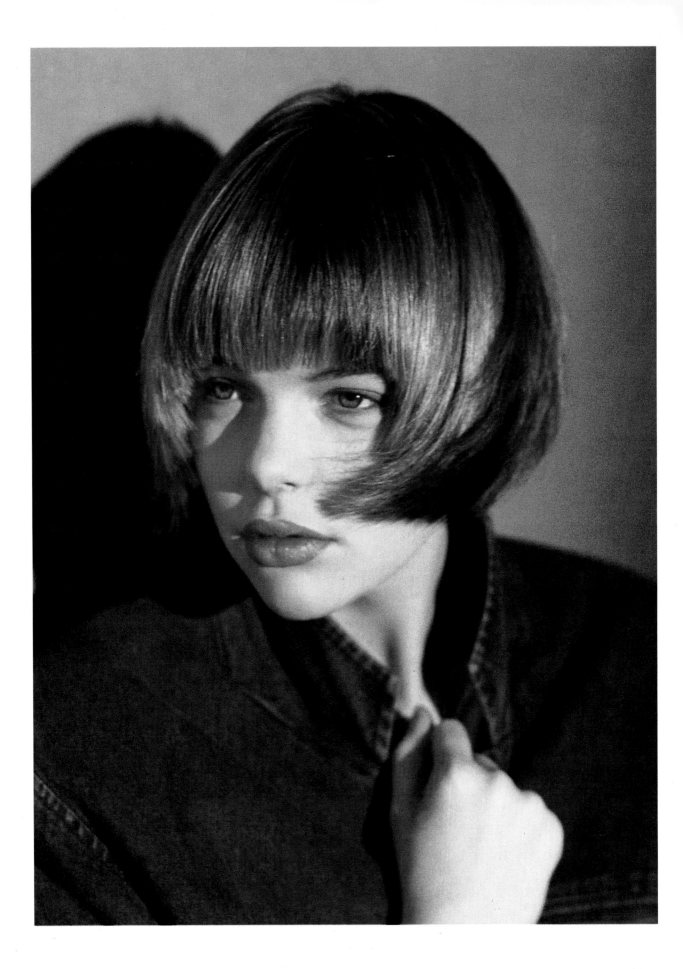

EMMA

◇ Emma's hair is naturally straight and very thick. It was highlighted with warm champagne lowlights and cut into a short, graduated bob which was brushed forward on to her cheeks.

○ Here we have a very natural, sporty look with little emphasis on any one particular feature.

Foundation A tinted moisturizer was used all over the face to act as a base.

Eyes A taupe eye shadow was brushed all over the eye, then a soft-brown liner was smudged along the upper eyelid and under the lower lashes.

Cheeks To give just a touch of colour to the cheek we added a pale-peach blusher.

Lips Chestnut lip gloss was applied and blotted to create a lip stain.

Denim is worn in both pictures. For day-time it is simple, for the evening the denim is dressed up with gold sequins.

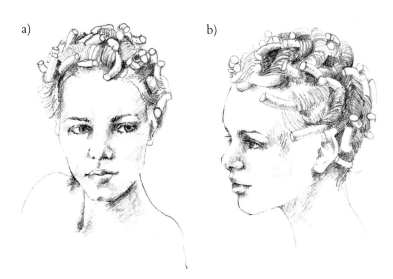

a)   b)

a) and b) A section of hair is rolled on to the Molton 'styler' backwards towards the scalp and the 'styler' is secured by bending the ends forward.

c) and d) A side view and a back view of the 'stylers' in place.

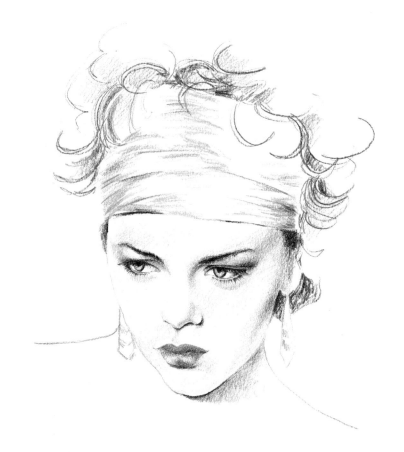

Foundation For the evening look, foundation was applied where needed, for example under the eyes or to cover any blemishes.

Eyes None of the day-time eye make-up was removed but the entire eyelid was simply brushed over with metallic gold eye shadow. The eyes were lined with cobalt-blue eye shadow and the same colour was used under the lower lashes and lightly smudged to avoid any hard lines. On the outer corners of the eyes we applied and smudged navy-blue pencil to create depth. Inside the eye, a line was made with cobalt-blue eye pencil.

Cheeks A blusher, which was a russet shade with a gold fleck, was applied over the existing one.

Lips On the lips, a lipstick of deeper russet than the blusher was applied and blotted. On top of this, gold iridescent was dabbed in the centre of the lower lip then blended using a finger.

◇ To transform Emma's hair for evening we set it in 'stylers'. A gold scarf was then wrapped around her forehead allowing the hair to tumble freely over it.

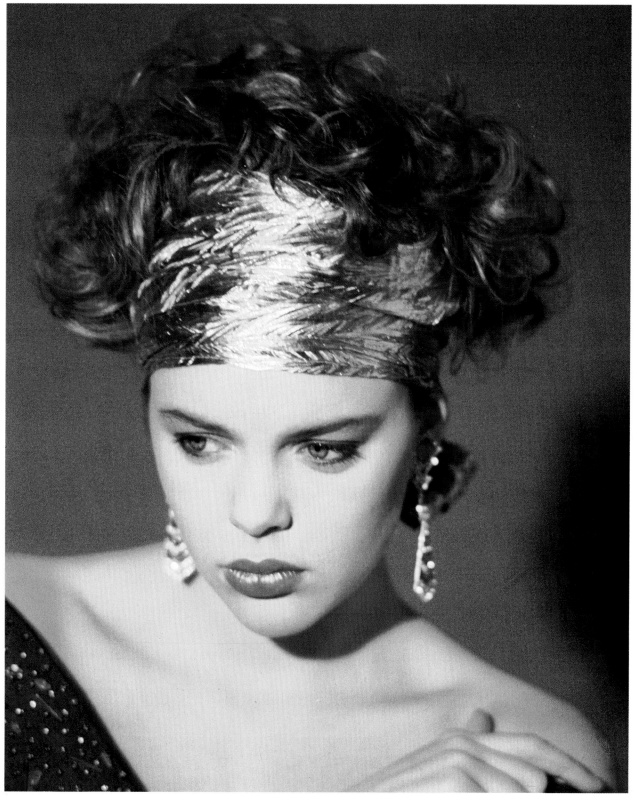

○ Here we used rich, jewelled colours such as amethyst,
sapphire and topaz.

From Day to Evening in Ten Minutes

Converting your day-time make-up to a mood suitable for the evening is less complicated than you might imagine. There is certainly no need to start all over again as the following procedure explains:

● Spray the face lightly with a mist of water or toner and then pat it dry with a tissue to remove any excess water.
● Tidy up under the eyes with a cotton bud. Freshen and even up the areas that need it with foundation. Then, lightly dust the face with powder.

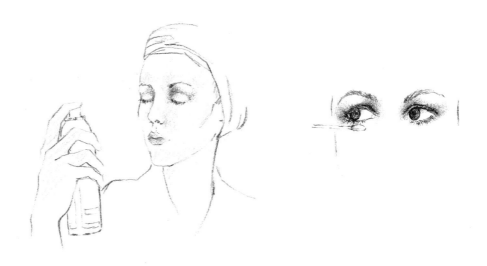

● Go over existing eye shadow and make it stronger and darker. This is the ideal moment to use an iridescent powder. It will give you a wonderfully delicate shimmer, so perfect for evening. Now re-define the eyes along the base of the lashes using either a soft-black or smoky-grey pencil.

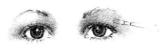

● Re-apply mascara. This is just the moment to try out some of the new coloured ones! Re-apply blusher.

● Choosing either your day-time lip colour or a darker shade of lip gloss, re-apply your lipstick. Then you can add a gold or silver metallic iridescent to your lips. Dab it on top of your existing lipstick with the tip of your finger. (*Iridescent* is loose, metallic powder, usually made out of mica. The powder is blended into a multitude of colours.)

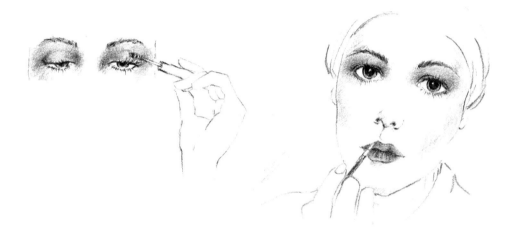

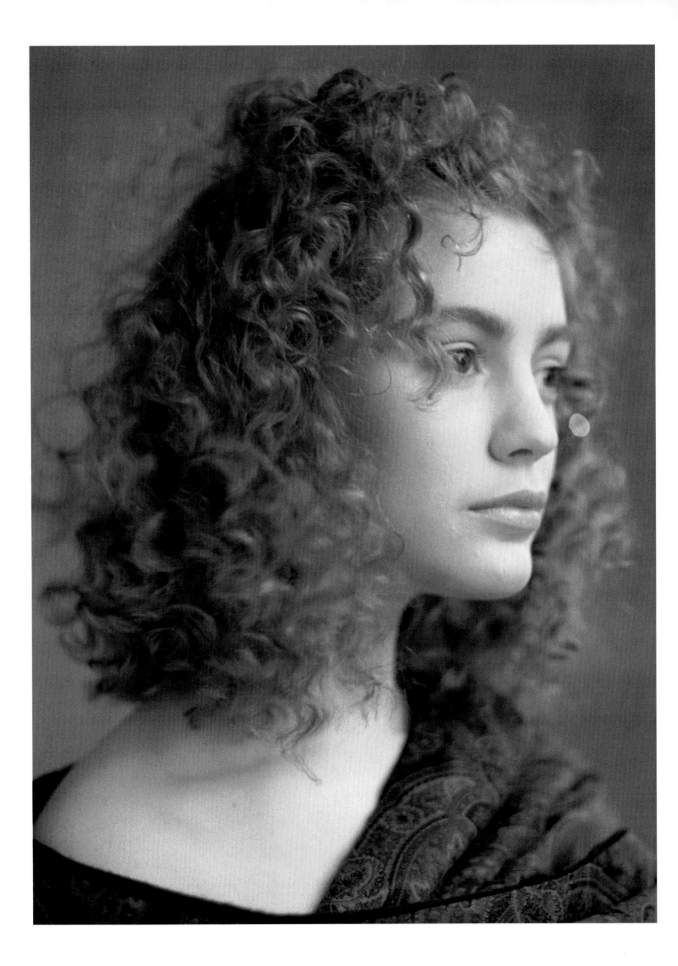

ELEONOR

◇ Eleonor's hair is dark blonde, and naturally straight and thick. It was set in Molton Browners to give this soft, natural look. Even though Eleonor has naturally straight hair, her own softness suggests an affinity with this look and style. We have let Eleonor's hair outline the features of her face and the soft wisps of curl follow the contours of her nose and mouth. Her hair-style relates to the features, the lines and the angles of her face making her look soft and feminine, and bringing out her natural beauty.

○ A creamy, ivory base was put all over the face and lightly dusted with translucent powder. The eyebrows were shaped and brushed. A rose-beige shadow was brushed all over the eye and a warm, soft brown put into the socket line from the inner corner to the outer edge of the eye and blended upwards. The upper lashes were lined with the same soft brown and smudged with a cotton bud to soften the line. On the lower lashes, soft-brown shadow was smudged dry from the outer corner of the eye to about three quarters of the way along. An earth-brown mascara was applied to the top lashes only. Muted rose blusher was dusted on the cheeks and the same colour in lipstick was brushed on to the lips and blotted. Finally a soft gold gloss was put on top of the lipstick, and blotted again to liven up the lipstick.

TRICHOLOGY

Trichology is the study of hair and originates from the word 'trichos', which is Latin for hair. There are three basic types of hair: Caucasian (European); Chinese/Japanese; Afro.

The Caucasian (European) type of hair is not quite straight and it may take many varied forms. When you wash Caucasian hair, choose a good conditioner that can be left on the middle length and on the ends of the hair, and not washed out; this will help to retain moisture.

The Chinese/Japanese type hair is dead straight, and as a result many people prefer to have it permed. This tends to dry the hair out, so it must be conditioned each time it is washed and given a conditioning treatment every four weeks or so.

Afro type hair tends to feel woolly, because of its tight curls. The scalp needs more looking after as it has a tendency to dry out. The best thing to use for this is a moisturizing scalp cream. With this particular type of hair a conditioner or oil should be left in the hair. This type of hair does not need to be washed too often; but it can benefit greatly from being conditioned between shampoos. Do this by applying a conditioner, leaving it on and then rinsing it off.

HAIR PROBLEMS
Your hair could be described as a barometer of your state of health. The two most obvious and common hair problems are: hair that is too dry and hair that is too oily and lank.

Oily hair is caused by too much sebum (natural oil) and the condition can be helped by diet. Therefore try to avoid fried or fatty foods, carbohydrates (e.g. chocolates and sweets) and spicy foods. There is a tendency to wash oily hair more often; if you do so, use a very mild shampoo and try to condition the ends of the hair at least once a week, otherwise they may become dry. As you may be washing your hair more often, be careful how you dry it. If you use a dryer, continue until the hair is three quarters dry, then leave it to finish itself off. This leaves some moisture for the hair to re-absorb.

Dry hair is caused by a number of things: frequent washing with a strong shampoo; hair drying with a dryer which is too hot; heated appliances; highlights and perms.

SCALP PROBLEMS

There are a number of scalp problems, most of them being various flaking or scaling disorders. There are about twenty of these and they are all generally referred to as dandruff. The term dandruff was invented by the American shampoo manufacturers in the 1920s, to describe a range of conditions that their particular shampoo might be designed to treat.

The most usual flaking disorders come under the following categories:

True or simple dandruff is a dry flaking scalp or scurf.

Waxy dandruff is seen as patches of yellowish, waxy flaking around the hairline or in patches on the head.

Oily dandruff shows itself as a diffuse, greyish, fine flaking often associated with hair loss. All these conditions may be attributed, in part, to poor diet or stress. It is always advisable to consult your doctor or a trichologist in the case of any persistent scalp disorders or hair loss.

USING A BLOW-DRYER

Many people blow dry their hair every time they wash it. However, if it is not done carefully it can cause damage. It is a myth that a powerful hair-dryer held close to the head will speed up the drying process. Time can often be saved by towel drying before blow drying.

You do not need the most powerful hair-dryer, and it should be held no closer than 10 cm (4 in) away from the head. At Molton Brown, we often hold a dryer as far away from the head as 15–23 cm (6–9 in). To test for the correct distance and heat, try the dryer on the back of your hand. The correct temperature will feel more like a warm Mediterranean breeze than a hot, Saharan-desert storm.

Another danger while blow drying is the misuse of your brush. Pulling the hair too harshly can be extremely damaging.

DENISE

◇ Denise has wonderful elfin features. In order to give volume, the hair was lifted repeatedly while it was being finger dried. The sides were cut and highly graduated into the ears, and the fringe was cut short to emphasize her petite features. Her long, slender neck is enhanced by the low 'v' of her dress.

○ Here is a symphony of golds and blues! The gold picks up the warmth of the hair and the blue on the eyelids reflects the earrings and dress. The emphasis is on the eyes and the fringe with a minimum of colour on the cheeks and lips.

Thick, Wavy Hair

WASHING AND DRYING

Thick, wavy, auburn hair has a tendency to be dry. It is best to towel dry it to remove the surface moisture before blow drying or finger drying the hair. Medium-length hair will need to be lifted up from the roots when it is dried with a blow-dryer.

If you want to wear this type of hair straight then, when you are drying it, use a brush and the hair-dryer together. In this way you will be gently lifting and straightening the hair without pulling it.

Very short, thick, wavy hair can be dried just by running your fingers through it. If you use a hair-dryer it will need to be lifted with both the hands and fingers as you dry it.

CUTTING

This kind of hair worn long can be left to hang straight down the back, but to soften the outline you can either cut a light fringe or allow a few strands to hang down round the face. If a fringe is cut it may need to be lightened by feathering it. Try to avoid pulling the hair back and just

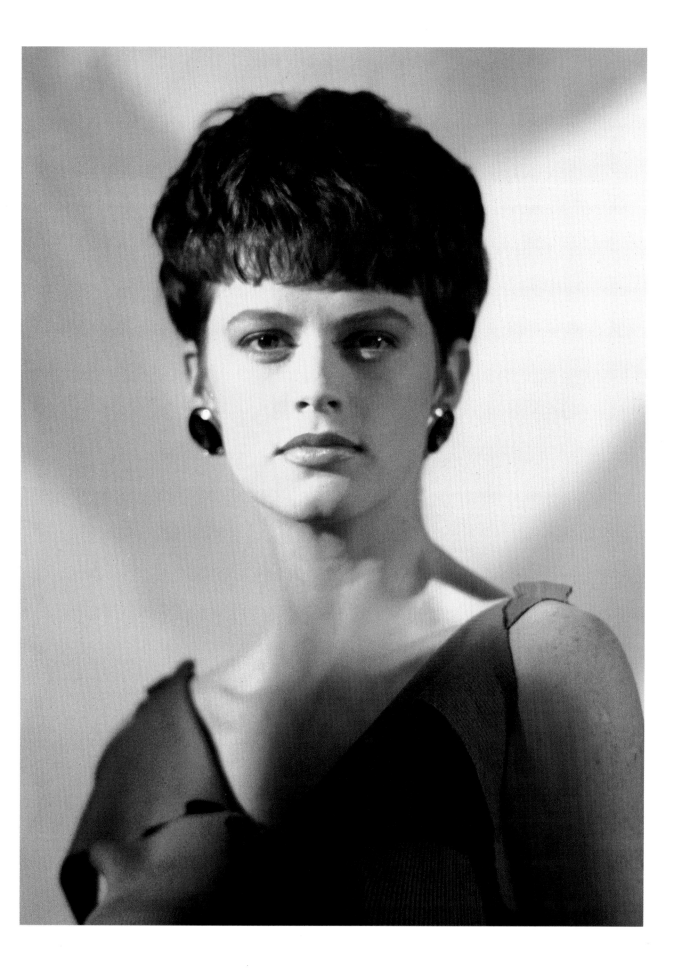

FELICITY

◇ Felicity's hair was brushed down across her forehead and completely taken back at the sides, creating this powerful look.

○ This effect is simple, but has a very strong impact. All the emphasis is on Felicity's fabulous lips with a minimum of make-up on her eyes. Her lips are outlined with a natural pencil following their original shape, then filled in with a metallic bronze lipstick. This was then blotted to remove the shine.

(Continued from p. 92)

tucking it behind the ears. If long hair is cut too quickly it can end up looking thick and lumpy. Medium-length hair can be graduated, but the graduation needs to be done very carefully otherwise it will look rather heavy.

Short hair of this sort can be cut very short if it suits your face. This hair has a lot of movement in it but would also need a lot of feathering to lighten it. If you have a fringe cut you will need to leave some of the hair longer and have it feathered.

SETTING
Long hair will set very well but will drop very quickly because of its weight. Remember to put very small sections of hair round each of the rollers or Molton Browners.

Medium-length hair will hold the set much better, but set small sections of hair at a time.

Very short hair does not need setting although the longer pieces, such as the fringe, respond well to gel.

HIGHLIGHTING AND TINTING
These processes make the hair drier so it will need constant conditioning and treatments to maintain its healthy appearance. This type of hair responds very well to being permed as it accentuates the natural movement of the hair.

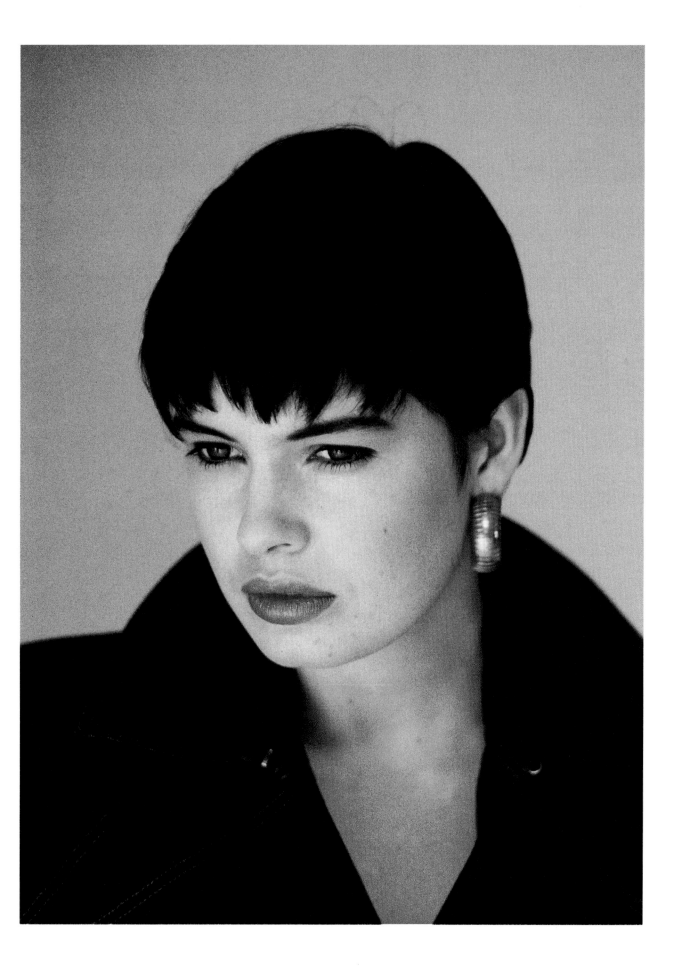

◇ The mood here is very much related to shadow and to the theme of light and dark. The dark hair is very strong and solid in contrast to the face. Deep graduation of the hair can lighten it and at the same time project a dreamy quality.

○ Felicity's eyes have been kept very simple in order not to detract from the feathery hair-line. The main emphasis is on her beautifully-shaped lips which were outlined with a fuchsia lip pencil and filled in with fuchsia lipstick.

Thick, Straight Hair

WASHING AND DRYING

You can shampoo thick, straight hair every day if you wish, but condition it well with a light conditioner. Wash it once only and do not use too much shampoo. Rinse it thoroughly to make sure that no shampoo is left in the hair before you condition it.

If your hair is long, thick and straight and you use a hair-dryer to dry it, then give it plenty of lift and hold the dryer well away from the head. This type of hair takes a long time to dry.

With medium-length and short hair, the hair needs to be lifted and given a lot of movement during the drying process.

CUTTING

The cut is very important with thick straight hair because it is so clearly seen. It is best to use any features that the hair has and to work with them. Particular features, such as a 'cowslick', a 'double crown', a 'widow's peak' or a 'duckstail' are very often found with this kind of hair. A bob suits thick, straight hair because it will hold both the shape and the set well. A style to avoid with medium-length hair of this sort is a graduated cut because the hair cannot hold the height and volume needed by this style to look good. In general it is best if this type of hair is kept either short and crisp, or simply long.

SETTING

If you want to be sure that your hair will stay set and looking the way you like it, then a perm would be the best solution. If you want to set your hair for a particular occasion, then do it lightly with the understanding that it will not last long.

Medium-length and shorter hair will hold a set better and the set will help give the hair height and volume. The way you set your hair should emphasize the shortness and crispness of the hair-cut. The hair holds much better if you use setting lotions and gels.

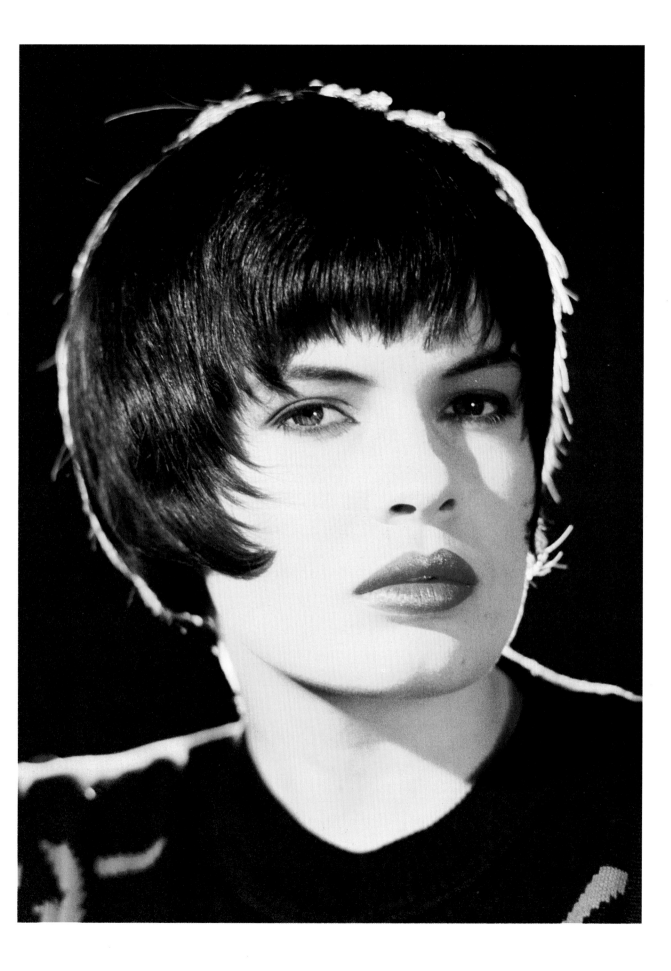

MIMI

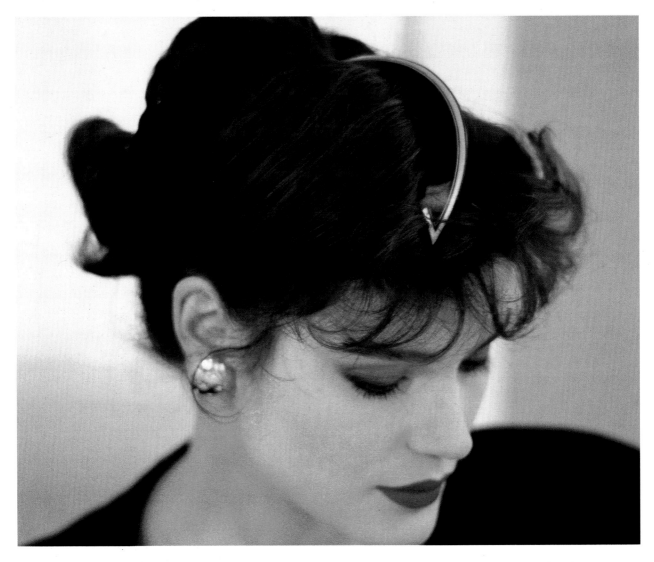

◇ Mimi's hair has been put up into three French pleats, one at the back and one at each side. The side pleats are held up by a pair of antique French combs.

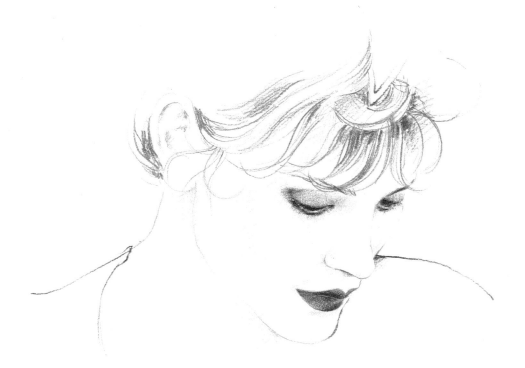

Eyes The eyebrows were shaped and defined using an eyebrow brush and feathering on brown eye shadow. Pale-ivory powder eye shadow was brushed over the entire eye area to act as a base. Dark brown eye shadow was brushed on the lid which was then lined with black eye pencil. Next, the outer corner of the eye was emphasized with black eye shadow which was smudged back along the lid over the black eye liner in order to create a smoky effect. The same was done under the lower lashes, but only three quarters of the way along. Black mascara was applied to the top lashes only.

Cheeks Nearly-nude blusher was used to emphasize the shape of the cheeks.

Lips The lips were first lined with red lip pencil and then filled in with midnight-red lipstick which was blotted and powdered.

○ Mimi's pale skin allows the emphasis to rest on the eyes and lips. Dark, smoky eyes and strong, matt-red lips combine with a hint of blusher to finish a classic look.

a)

b)

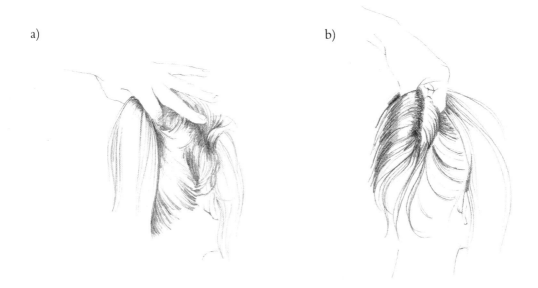

The hair has been divided into two sections: front and back.

a) The back is taken up and held in a pony tail.

b) The pony tail is then twisted by a twist of the thumb into a French pleat, leaving a few strands to hang down naturally.

c)

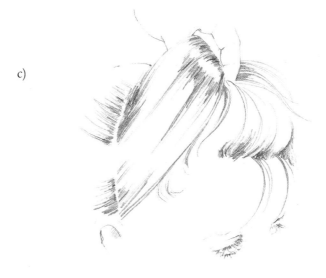

c) The same French pleat twist movement is used on the front section of the hair, which is then held in place by an antique comb.

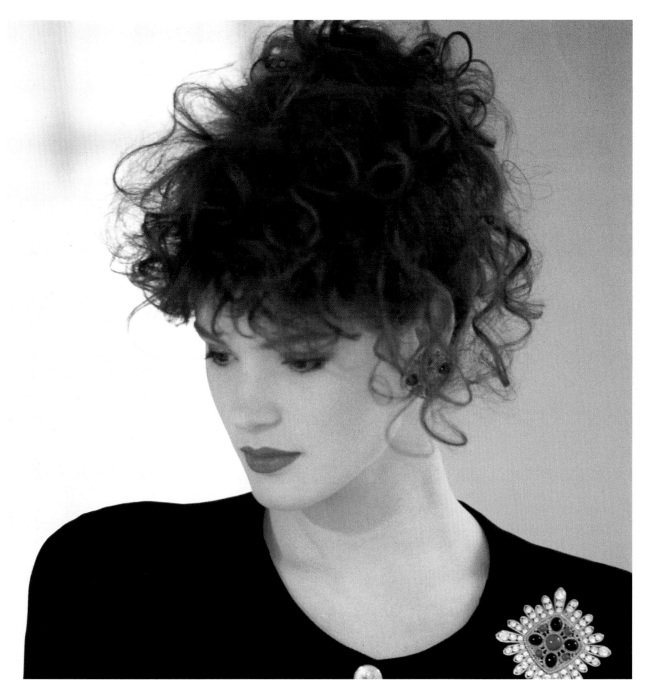

◇ The hair was completely set in half-inch Molton Browners. Even though the fringe is curled it still maintains its shape and the hair is allowed to fall lightly and freely round the sides of the face. The hair contrasts with Mimi's severe black dress which in turn sets off her brilliant pearl, ruby and jet brooch.

○ This classic, French look focuses on the dark, smoky eyes, very pale skin and strong, matt-red lips.

AKURA

◇ The vibrant blue, silk scarf that drapes Akura's body is swept up into her hair and held by the parrot comb. This also secures her hair while leaving a soft cascade to tumble down, like fine threads, each side of her face.

○ This is a beautiful, tropical look! Because Akura has dark skin she can carry vibrant colours without looking in the least bit garish.

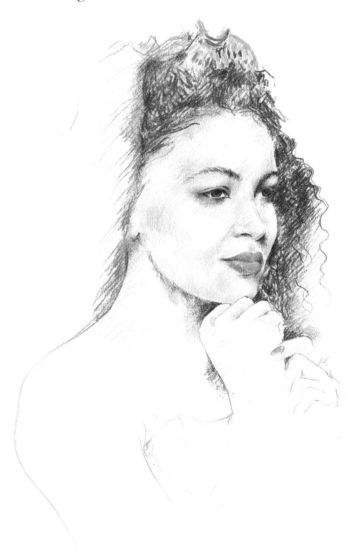

Here the focus is on the eyes and bright lips.

Eyes First, the eyebrows were brushed and shaped. Emerald-green eye shadow was applied, with a light hand, over the entire eye surface, and yellow eye shadow was added on the browbone. Electric-blue eye shadow, used wet as a liner, was drawn along the upper eyelid. For increased depth, the same eye shadow (this time used dry) was applied over the liner. Amethyst shadow was smudged just beneath the lower lashes and the final touch was made with purple mascara.

Cheeks and lips Nearly-nude blusher was swept over the cheeks, and on the lips we used a vibrant orange lipstick.

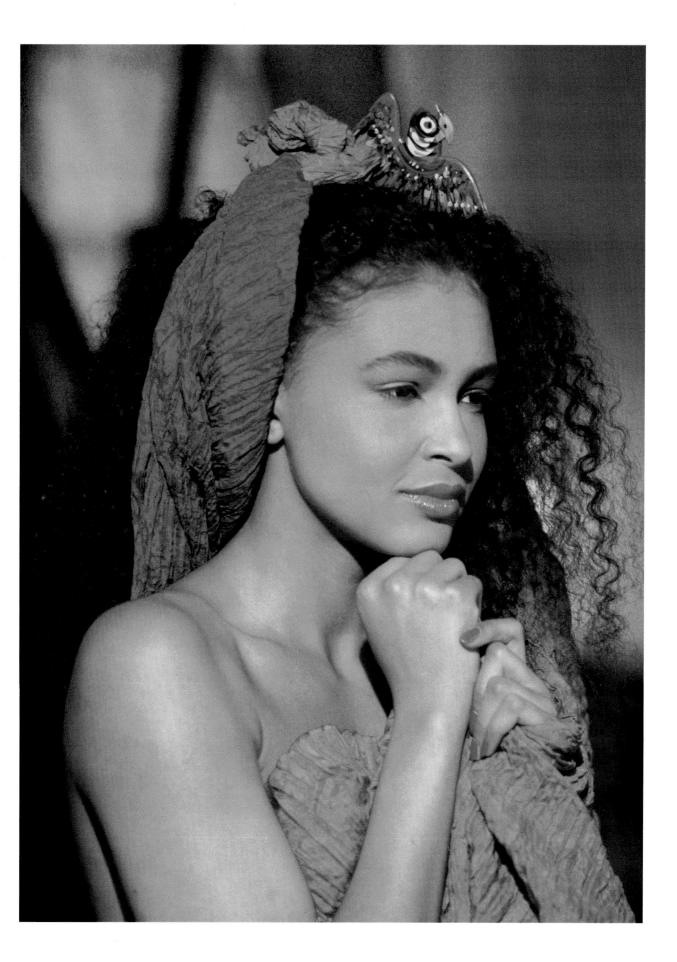

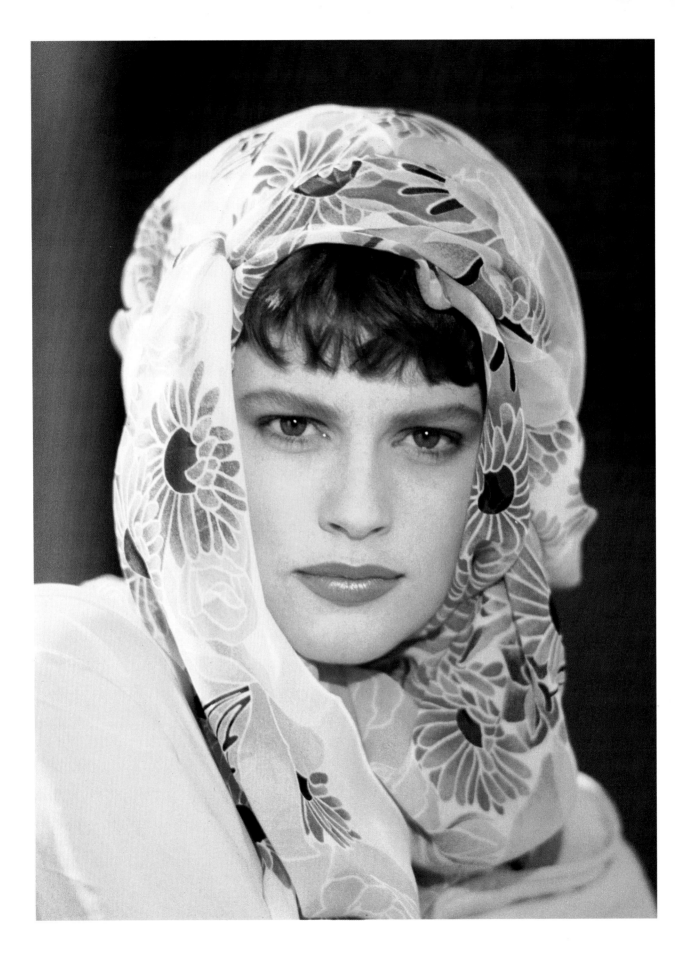

DENISE

○ This is an example of how you can effectively use multi-colours on the eyes. The secret is in the careful blending of the colours.

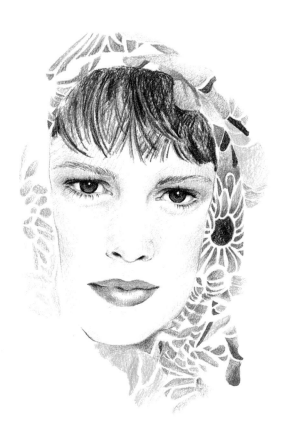

Foundation A foundation which matched Denise's skin tone was applied and followed by translucent powder lightly brushed all over the face.

Eyes Canary-yellow eye shadow was applied all over the eye to make a base and to act as a highlight. In the socket line an apricot shade of shadow acting as a highlight was added. On the upper eyelid, a royal-blue shadow was used wet, as an eye liner, then smudged to give a soft effect. Under the lower lashes, purple eye shadow was applied and lightly smudged.

Cheeks and lips A coral-pink blusher was used and a pink lip colour chosen for the lips.

The secret here is to blend all the colours carefully so that they merge into one another while retaining their separate identities.

PREPARING FOR SUMMER

Just when the tunnel of winter seems endless the days at last begin to lengthen, the leaves and blossoms appear and suddenly, the first warm rays of the sun fill us all with a new, refreshed energy. We react to this in many different ways: by spring-cleaning our homes, by doing the garden or by running to the shops to buy something new to wear. It is also a time when we take a good look at our bodies. We have probably put on a few extra pounds during the winter and now we instinctively feel the need to take more exercise, to be out in the fresh air, and to change our diet. The summer brings with it a new variety of fresh fruit and vegetables and it becomes easier to eat more healthily.

Spring is also the time to begin some gentle exercise; this may involve simply walking more or perhaps taking up jogging. If you do take up jogging make sure you use the correct shoes and try to do it in a park rather than on the hard pavements as the air is cleaner and the delights of the surroundings — the summer flowers and the trees — are more beneficial. If you live in the city, swimming becomes more attractive again and it is one of the best forms of all-round exercise you can have.

The approach of summer might tempt you to take a sauna. If you do, it will help you to thoroughly scrub away the winter dirt and dullness. If possible, take a whole day off and groom yourself for the summer days ahead. You will probably find that your legs and underarms need waxing or shaving and that your skin is generally quite dry and dull from all those winter months when it was hidden under clothes. If you can afford it, treat yourself to a facial, a manicure and a pedicure. Or, if you prefer, do these for yourself at home allowing yourself time to do them without skimping and rushing. Summer is a good time to take a new look at your hair and to decide whether it is the moment for a change; this may be a new hair-cut or a more adventurous step, for example adding highlights or lowlights. These will catch the sunlight and add reflected sparkle to your hair. You may also like to look at your hair accessories and invest in one of the new season's cotton headbands or the new range of bright elastics, bows or clips.

Finally, spring is the time to look at your make-up. Organize a clear-out and wash your favourite make-up bag. The range of colours that looked fine for winter may now have a rather dull, severe appearance when worn against summer clothes. Take a good look at the new season's colours, at the clothes you have, and at any new ones that you have bought; you may find that all you need is a new lipstick, or a bright-coloured mascara, and possibly an iridescent for summer evenings.

Sun Care

We all feel healthier when we have a golden tan, but great care must be taken to achieve it safely.

Firstly, before the start of your holiday, prepare the skin by lavish application of a rich moisturizer. Skin that is dry is already being shed, and exposure to the sun will only speed up this process. Use a lotion with a high S.P.F. factor at the start of your holiday and as the skin becomes acclimatized, progress to a lower S.P.F. factor. It is important to be patient. It takes three days to activate the melanin within the skin, so prolonged sunbathing in the first few days only results in burning.

To protect the hair, particularly permed, tinted and highlighted hair, make use of a specially formulated hair lotion which contains a sun filter. This will prevent the hair from becoming dry and lifeless, and eases combing after swimming.

Summer Make-up

During the summer, your make-up will complement and blend with your tan, that is if you have one. If you don't, then use a tinted moisturizer which will give your face a glow.

Use neutral colours on your eyes in the summer and put all the emphasis on your lips. Here, you can use really strong colours such as fuchsia, bright mango, pink and red. These look best when set off by a tan.

Instead of using eye shadow, try a coloured mascara for a lovely effect.

In hot weather, keep your blusher to a minimum. Your skin colour will come through and give a lovely glow to your cheeks.

All summer colours should be sheer rather than opaque. Sheer colours are light and fresh which is what you need at this time of year.

a) Sometimes an iridescent eye shadow, when used very sparingly, can look lovely, simply because it is very sheer.

Here a gold eye shadow was lightly dusted all over the eye, then a copper shade was used on the lid and continued a little way along the lower lash. Black mascara was used on the eyelashes, and a hint of natural blusher was brushed on the cheeks. The focus is on the lips which are fuchsia pink; a very sheer lipstick was used so that the lips show through it.

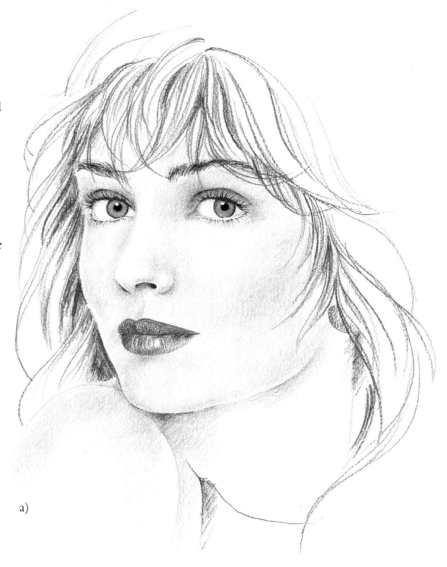

a)

b) In summer, a strong line of bright colour can be very effective. You can line the upper lid at the base of the eyelashes and smudge it gently with your finger so that it does not look too hard. We have used a bright blue, but other shades, such as purple and lime-green, can also look stunning. To complete the look, we have kept the cheeks very soft. The lips can be very strong, but in order to keep all the emphasis on the eyes, here we chose a very sheer pink lipstick touched with a gold fleck.

b)

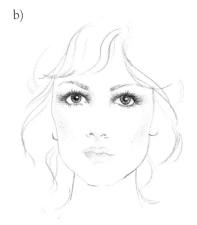

c) This is a monochromatic look which means that we are using one colour, in a range of different tones, for all the make-up on the face. In this case, the theme colour is bronze.

Bronze eye shadow is lightly dusted over the eyelid which is then lined with a soft-brown pencil, softly smudged to finish.

The mascara is brown, the cheeks have a copper-tone blusher on them and the lips have a copper lipstick.

c)

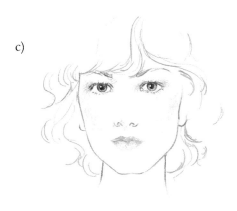

d)

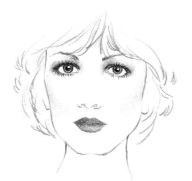

d) This is more of a summer-evening look than a day-time one. We have made the eyes smoky by using charcoal grey rather than black. The cheeks are lightly dusted with burnt-orange blusher and for the lips we selected a sheer, orange-red lipstick.

In all these summer make-ups, the skin shows through because powders and lipsticks are very sheer and contain just a hint of colour.

WINTER SKIN-CARE AND MAKE-UP

In winter, our skin's renewing process becomes sluggish as the weather gets colder. The greatest danger to our skin at this time of year is our own laziness and reluctance to look after our skin properly: our bodies spend much of the time covered up; we feel less inclined to remove clothes and take exercise; and we often neglect our diet.

As winter progresses you may start to notice dry patches on your face and body. The cold, combined with the wind, can destroy the skin's small blood vessels which are then called broken capillaries. But it is the dryness of the wind that causes the most problems, for example, chapping, wrinkles, and premature ageing of the skin. All skins suffer from the ravages of winter, even oily skin.

Protection is your best line of defence. At this time of year it is even more important to give time and attention to your face; it is a good time to have a professional facial. Continue your usual cleansing routine and supplement it regularly with a home facial, steam, and scrub. After cleansing and toning it is essential to use a moisture retainer on your face, followed by your usual moisturizer. A moisture retainer is a blend of natural sugars and amino acids which adds moisture to your skin. A moisturizer simply seals in the moisture which is actually present.

Outdoor activities, whether it be a brisk walk in the park or skiing in the mountains, are wonderfully invigorating. However, do remember to give yourself that extra protection of a good sun-screen and a lip salve or lip balm because although the sun may not feel hot, the U.V.B. rays are still present.

In winter, being indoors can be just as hard on your skin. Dry air from central heating can rob skin of moisture and make it feel parched. Keeping a dish of water in your bedroom or office, or using a humidifier, can help. Always use a moisturizer regardless of your skin type, and if you have dry skin a richer night cream can help.

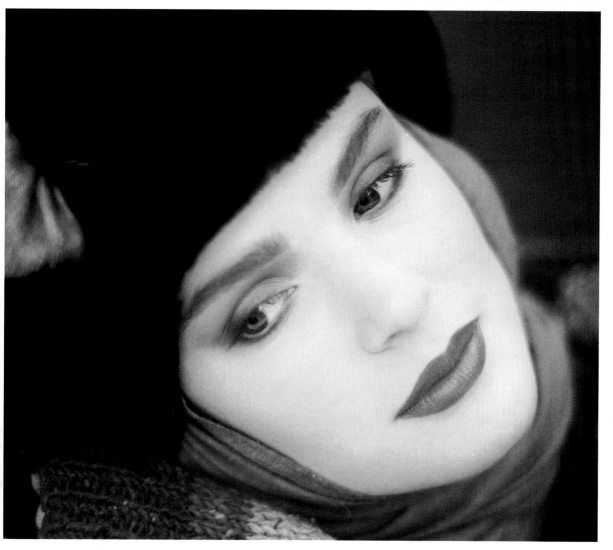

○ A pale-ivory foundation was used and then translucent powder was brushed all over the face. The eyebrows were brushed and shaped. A pale-brown-rose shadow was brushed all over the eye and then a dark-burgundy-brown was brushed along the base of the upper lashes and blended upward to meet the lighter eye shadow. The same burgundy colour was used as an eye liner and also brushed along the lower lashes. A very pale-pink ivory was then used as a highlight just under the eyebrows. To finish a red-earth-brown mascara was used on both the upper and lower lashes. A soft-rose blusher was lightly brushed onto the cheeks. On the lips, we used a strong, terracotta lipstick which was brushed on and then blotted in keeping with the matt effect that is a feature of this winter look.

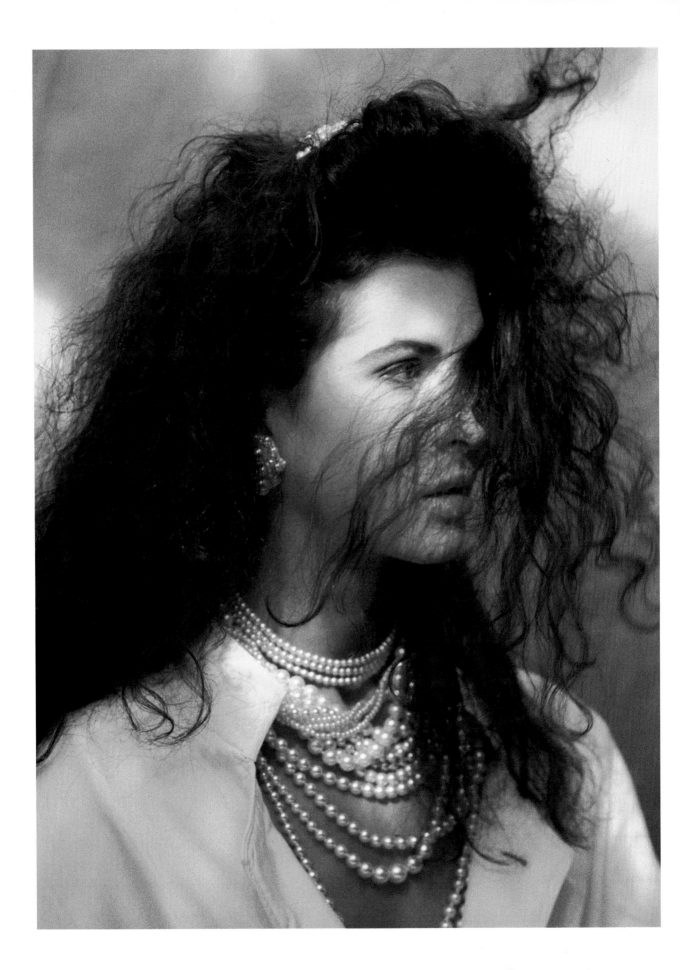

STEPHANIE

◇ Stephanie projects a poetical mysterious mood with her hair gently thrown across her face. The contrast created by sweeping the hair away from the face and then allowing it to fall back highlights the strength of her features.

○ The make-up reflects the cascade of pearls she is wearing. There is a pearly finish on her eyes and a pearl lip gloss on the lips. The lips were blotted so that the glossiness was removed and just the shimmer remained. No blusher was used.

Fine, Wavy Hair

WASHING
Fine, wavy hair needs a special kind of care and attention. In particular it benefits from careful washing because if it is not absolutely clean the hair tends to look lank and the ends can look dry and split, especially if it is long. It is essential, therefore, to wash fine hair frequently and to condition it lightly every time you wash it. Once a week you should use a heavier conditioner on your hair.

DRYING
Fine hair dries very quickly unless it is highly processed, for example, by tinting, perming, or straightening. If you use a blow dryer, remember to towel dry your hair first to remove the worst of the moisture and then to hold the dryer well away from the hair. If your hair is short then finger drying is an excellent method to use as it will help to contain the hair's tendency to frizz. It will also give volume and height to hair, where this is needed.

CUTTING

If you have fine hair you need a style that is heavy and chunky so that the hair is not thinned and made to look lank. If your hair is long it will respond to gentle graduation. If it is curly it can be cut very short and would look marvellous if it were cut to just an inch all over. Medium-length hair has a tendency to rise up and look shorter, so if you like your hair to look a certain length then make sure that the cut is a little longer than you think you want it.

If you have a round face, take particular care over the length of your hair. If it is cut to the wrong length it will emphasize the 'roundness' of your appearance. If you have a long, slender face the hair can look unflattering if it is left too long, because it will exaggerate this feature.

SETTING AND FINISHING

If your hair is very curly it will set quickly, so you will find Molton Browners or large heated rollers the best way to finish your hair. It is important not to over-set fine hair, so when you are about half-way through fixing them check on the first rollers to see how the hair is taking.

Fine hair tends to go frizzy and hazy and reacts badly to being brushed, especially if it is long. It is best to use a wide-toothed comb and your fingers, as well as a brush, to keep the hair under control and to stop too much static accumulating.

When cut to the right length, short, fine hair can be left to dry naturally and is one of the easiest kinds of hair to manage.

◇ Stephanie's hair was swept up and pulled through a cone that had been wrapped in raffia to match her dress. The ends were left to fall naturally down around her neck.

○ When the hair is really strong then the make-up must be simple. Here is an uncluttered make-up which does not detract from the hair.

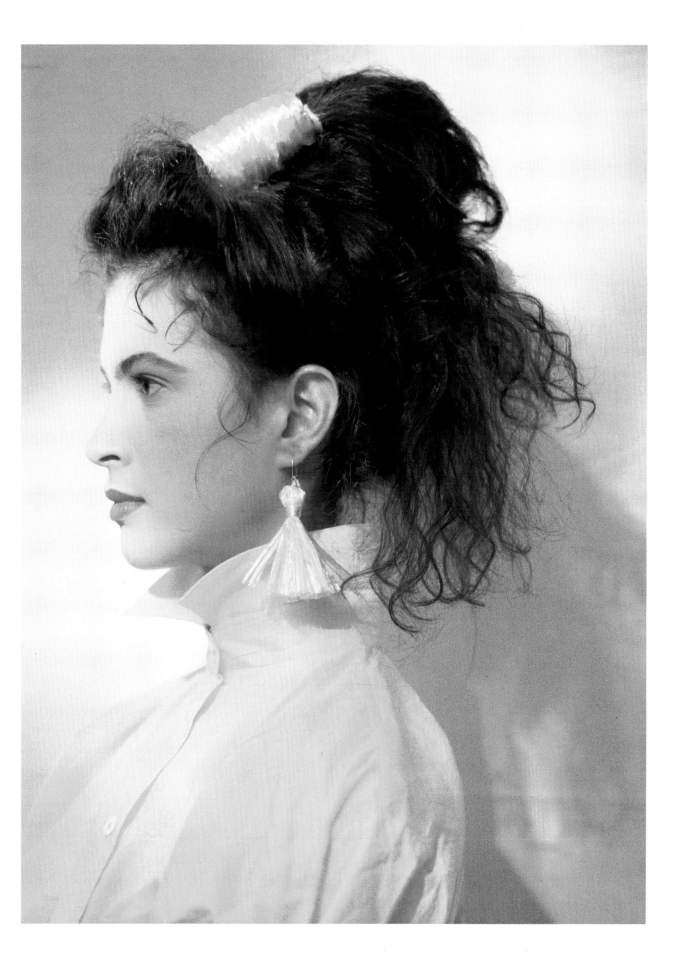

DEBBIE

◇ Debbie's hair is long and has strong movement, and the way it is put up and bound together reflects this. Here, her hair was taken up and twisted into knots. An iridescent, crescent moon holds the hair in place, as well as reflecting the theme of her earrings and clothes.

○ A modern 'Victorian' look using gold, copper and black complements the jacket and accessories. The eyes were dusted with gold, and black shadow was added to the lids. Gold iridescent was lightly smudged under the lower lashes and black mascara applied to both upper and lower lashes. The cheeks were brushed with a gold-copper blusher. A bronze lipstick was used with a dab of gold powder smudged along the lower lip.

a) The hair is parted down the middle and one half of the hair is held and twisted in an anti-clockwise direction.

b) The hair gradually twists itself into knots. The ends of the hair are secured to the head with a grip.

a)

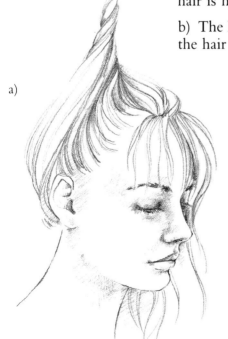

b)

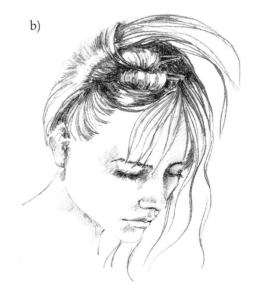

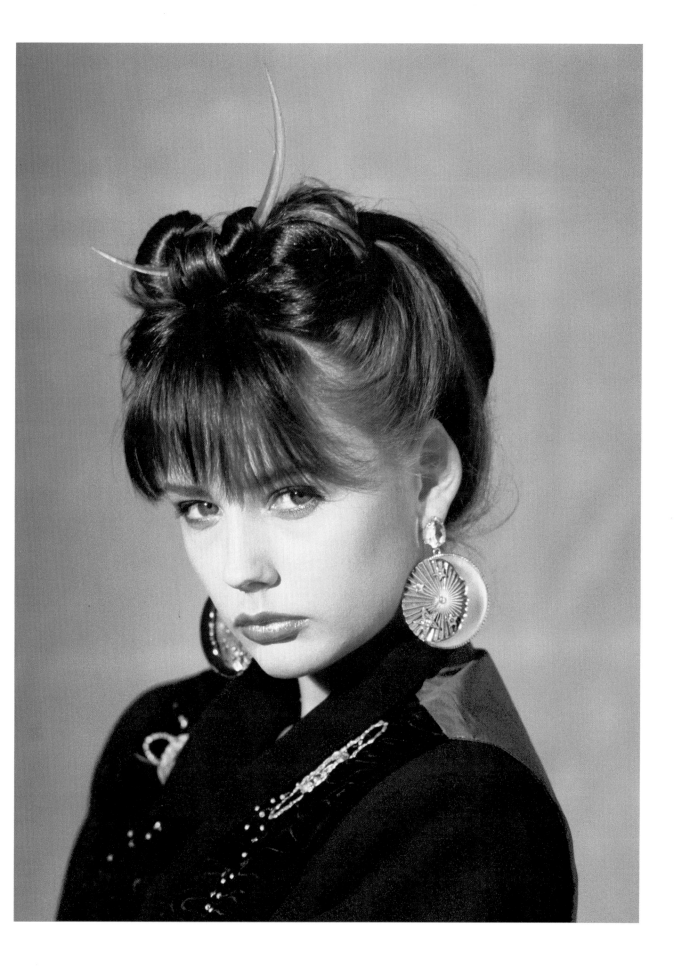

c) The remaining hair is taken and twisted using the same method, but in a clockwise direction.

d) The ends of the hair are fixed with pins before positioning slides or combs to complete the hair-style.

c)

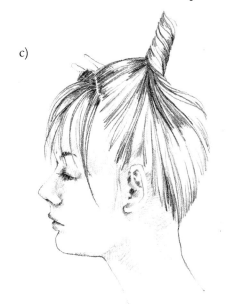

d)

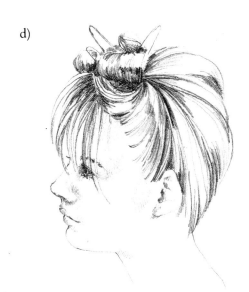

PUTTING UP HAIR

Throughout the ages women have always worn their hair up and have instinctively created beautiful ways of doing so. The style a woman chooses to dress her hair reflects the individual personality of the woman and the impression she wishes to project.

Hair can be put up in many different ways; by tying, twisting, curling, looping and plaiting, for example.

The basic chignon pin, whether it is simple or ornate, plastic or tortoiseshell, can provide a woman with endless permutations for pinning up her hair. With one carefully positioned pin, she can secure the hair firmly and look stunning. Elastic bands provide one of the easiest ways of putting up hair and, fortunately, today the bands are designed to be soft so that they do not split the hair. They also come in many wonderful colours.

There is no end of variety of tools and materials you can use to put up your hair. Slides, combs, scarves, ribbons and leather are some of the more obvious ones.

Choosing Accessories

Choice of accessories is always intimately linked with the woman who is wearing them. The way someone chooses and wears an accessory is completely individual and it will reflect something positive about that person. A woman will have a definite preference for the colour of her accessories, the texture and the quality of the material they are made of, and the kinds of beads or gems that decorate them. She will have an affinity with certain materials and colours and be unable to wear accessories that do not appeal to her.

Types of Accessories

Accessories for the hair come in a multitude of materials, colours, designs and textures. There are combs studded with beads, sequins, gems, stones and glass. There are slides made out of plastic, or metal such as titanium, steel, pure silver and gold. There are bands covered with cotton, silk, chiffon, velour, golden lurex, tie-and-dye, net and towelling. And for special occasions we have pearls, lace, and cream, silken flowers. There are pins, slides, combs, and bows with every kind of delicate or outrageous ornamentation. Finally, there is the original, metal or plastic hair pin and the traditional black silk bow.

An accessory has two functions: one is to hold the hair away from the face and to keep it in place; the other is to create a hair-shape that is flattering. The way in which the accessory is placed in the hair is vitally important and relates to the angle of the accessory in relation to the cut and set of the hair. The movement of the hair over the head is very important and must be taken into account when placing the accessory in the hair. It is the angle at which the hair lies across the head, combined with the movement of the hair and the total shape it creates, that will make an accessory look effective. Just as the cut of the hair will emphasize the good points of a woman's face so the accessory will add to both the cut and the set of the hair. The accessory should never contradict the hair style. Its function is to relate to the mood and the style of a woman by its form, its shape, and its design. The addition of these little features to the hair creates the total effect. The combination of them makes the whole effect either 'right' or 'wrong' and this effect is very individual. When it is right, we achieve what we are always looking for — the special effect. Accessories are rather like the particular flowers a woman loves or the perfume she wears. The hairdresser, by his or her intuitiveness, comes as near as possible to finding out what is right for each woman. A hairdresser will extend a woman's style and be just that little bit more daring than she herself might be. But in the end it will always be the woman's own instinctive feeling for what is 'right' that will make the accessory she chooses look stunning.

Accessorizing Techniques

It is endlessly fascinating and creative to vary and add interest to your usual hair-style by means of accessorizing. Some of the techniques are simple; others require time and practice. Consider the following ideas.

Hair crochet Secure the thread to the hair using a hair hook. Work up towards the centre of the head, continually looping the hair. Secure the hair by pulling the thread through the last loop several times.

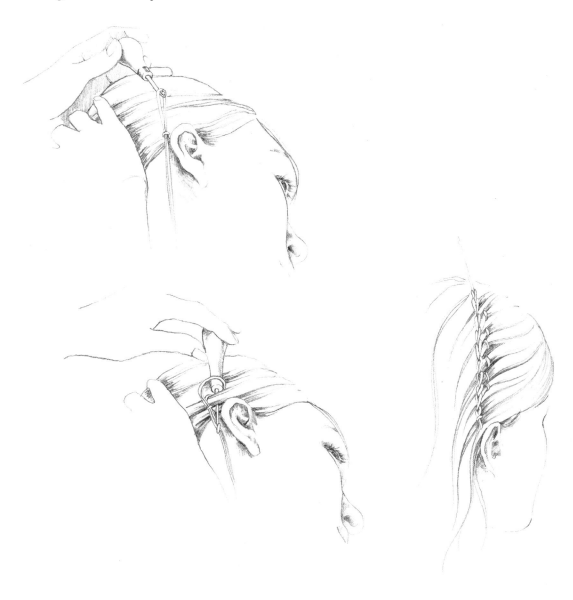

Putting in Combs Many people do not know how to put a comb in the hair, others complain that when they do it does not stay in place. Follow this procedure. Take up a section of your hair and fix it to the head with two grips facing in opposite directions and meeting in the middle. Place the comb just in front of and on top of the grips, to hide them.

The grips take the pressure away from the teeth of the comb and hold the hair so that the comb is not under strain. This helps to keep the comb in place. (The same method can be used for securing a slide.)

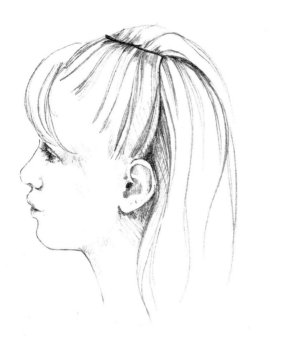
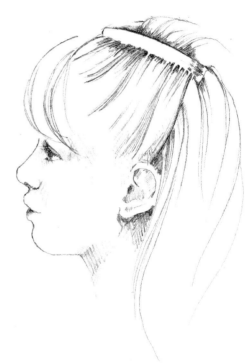

Binding Hair (see opposite) The front section of hair is twisted and held by a large clip. A length of thread is attached to a hair hook and the thread is then put into the hair and pulled through it. The hook goes through the loop and collects the ends of the thread bringing them back through the loop. This secures the thread around the hair.

Continue to make loops, collecting the ends and binding them around the hair. To finish, secure the hair by pulling the end of the thread through the same loop several times.

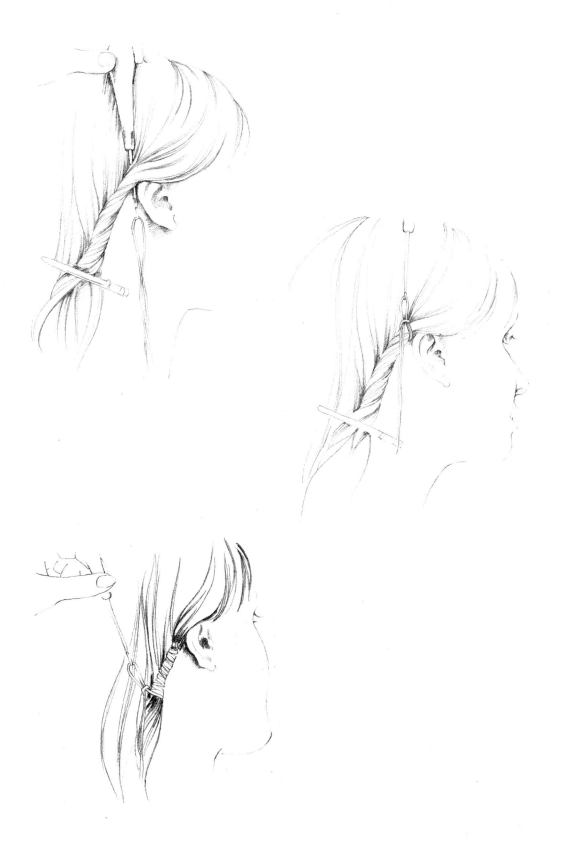

THE ALEXANDER TECHNIQUE

To help me towards living a healthy, balanced life I like to enjoy myself as fully as I can. I like to laugh as much as possible but not turn away from sorrow. I am happier when my body feels healthy and fit, so I walk, bicycle, eat and sleep well and practise the Alexander Technique.

The principle behind the Alexander Technique is choosing to respond to life by opening to it instead of reacting to life with contraction. This is not at all easy. We have been taught to react to life by being either defensive or aggressive. And we find ourselves, whether we wish it or not, behaving in habitual ways. How often do you say or feel, 'Oh, I wish I hadn't said that.' Or conversely, 'I wish I had been able to respond more freely?' Very often, we are caught in conflict and indecision, not knowing which way to turn.

The Alexander Technique gives you a moment of pause, a moment of choice, which can break through the habitual constricting patterns of behaviour. In a session with a teacher you are taught to be aware of your body and yourself as an integrated whole, in a quite new and very enjoyable way. Then you are helped to repeat this experience for yourself in daily life. Take, for example, a woman who is nervous and under pressure at work, or bored with not enough to do. She will contract her body and perhaps get a headache, back ache or other symptoms of discomfort. In her session with her teacher she will be taught to sit at her desk with the minimum of tension, to be aware of the positions of her head, neck and back and from these, to sense herself as an individual. The woman will be taken from standing to sitting, sitting to standing in a new and vivid way. This will help her to notice for herself that when her boss comes in she puts her head to one side and contracts her spine, or that she crosses her legs in a nervous and tense manner. And she will begin to be able to release herself from these habits.

I have found that people of all ages, not just the young

and relatively healthy, can be helped by the technique. Young children having difficulty adjusting to school, children with some physical handicap, people in their eighties needing help to straighten their spine can all benefit. At every age we are faced with different difficulties and may need help. Especially interesting are the times of teenage and menopause which, when handled rightly, are rich with possibilities for change, growth and flowering. Unfortunately, more often than not, they are times of dread!

At times, many of us are inclined to be too self-effacing and feel that we have to manage on our own, whereas a little professional assistance at the first signs of trouble, or even better before that, can save a lot of pain. It always astonishes me how many people accept that aching feet and legs are part of shopping, aching backs are part of ironing and headaches part of human relationships, without asking themselves if these discomforts are really necessary? Furthermore, why do they not see them as the first signs of misuse which, becoming chronic, could lead to illness or even surgery. Cars need regular maintenance and our bodies which are infinitely more subtle, delicate, complex and wonderful than a piece of machinery need similar care.

In our present society we are constantly being thrown off balance. We may lose ourselves in violent over-activity for a while and then collapse in a sludge. We may be surrounded by too many people one day, and suffer alone in unwanted solitude, the next day. We may take a lot of exercise at the weekends and then spend the week in stuffy offices and cramped conditions. Our relationships with others are seldom stable and supportive. So in the end we are left with only one possibility: that of bettering our relationship with ourselves. With the help of the Alexander Technique, a sense of well-being can be attained that makes us less dependent on external circumstances. Each of us has an innate sense of balance, but we often need help and encouragement to find it. When we do, then quite a new and exciting independence and joy in life can be ours!

Diana Dante

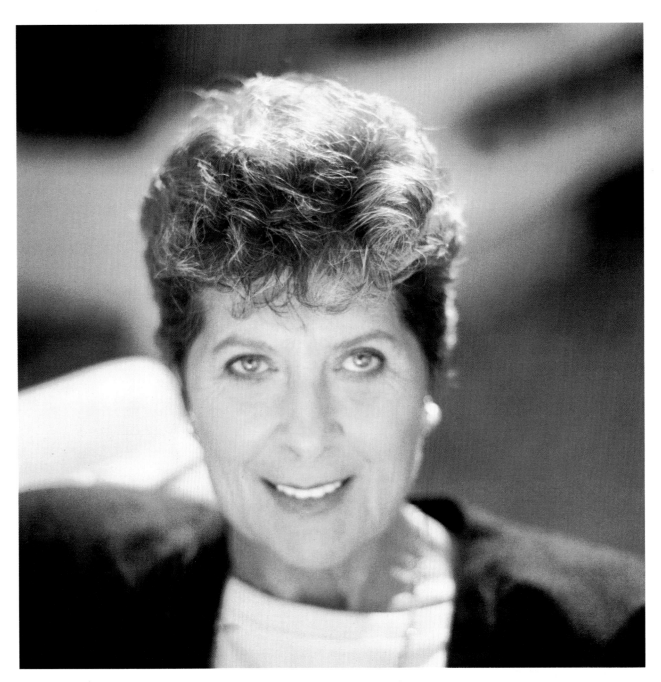

1. Day-time look

◇ The hair was cut short at the sides and left longer on top using the natural curl to give volume and softness. The colour is natural, proving how very attractive grey streaks can be. The haircut reflects the woman's strong, determined and youthful features.

○ A soft, beige shadow was used all over the eye with Silver Dawn on the lid, and navy smudged around the eye. On the cheeks we used terracotta blusher and on the lips London brick.

THE OLDER WOMAN

As a woman grows older she has to face all sorts of subtle changes, her hair being but one of them. Very few women escape going grey to some degree and they are then faced with deciding whether to live with it or change it. This is where a trusted hairdresser and colourist can be a great support.

Thanks to the great advances in hair colouring, today women can hide their grey subtly with products which look beautifully natural and do not harm their hair. It is a mistake to try to make your hair the same colour as it was when you were younger, because over the years your skin tone has also changed. If you do decide to change your hair colour then try to do it in gradual stages as there is always the problem of regrowth to contend with.

Try to keep the cut of your hair simple and the colouring subtle. This does not mean that you cannot experiment.

For older women who are, quite naturally, concerned about their appearance, perhaps the most useful make-up guideline is 'less is more'. As you age, your skin-care routine may need to be adjusted. Regardless of skin type you may notice that your skin is drier than it was when you were in your thirties. It is vital to make sure that the cleanser you use is extremely gentle and the toners not too harsh. It is a myth that women, as they grow older, should use a heavier moisturizer. It should of course be rich, but at the same time it should feel light to the touch and it should not leave the skin surface feeling greasy. At night, if you wish, you can add an eye cream, a neck cream and a night cream to your skin-care routine. Here again, be careful not to use heavy products as there is a danger of the skin becoming too dependent on them.

As we get older it is wise to avoid heavy make-up because, instead of hiding lines, it accentuates them even more. During the day, all that is needed is a light-weight foundation — this should also be used as a concealer which can be applied to areas that need more coverage. (The normal type of concealer is too heavy and makes wrinkles look more pronounced, particularly around the eyes.) After the foundation, apply just a light dusting of powder. Too much powder is also ageing.

When making up the eyes, again, it is important to be light-handed. Avoid brash colours, but also avoid the brown range as this tends to make one look tired. A good, neutral, everyday colour would be grey or soft navy. You may prefer to use a cream eye shadow, but if so, remember to use an eye-shadow fixative, otherwise the cream will end up in the wrinkles around the eyes. When deciding on mascara, a black or dark navy is nice, but again, avoid dark brown.

For blusher, a powder terracotta shade is good, as it is both neutral and warm. However, this certainly does not mean that you should feel restricted to this shade. You may prefer to use a blusher in a cream form.

When making up the lips, don't be afraid of bright, bold colours! Neutral shades are fine, but the bold ones liven up the whole face. Keep away from soft, pastel colours because these tend to look very bland on an older face.

In the evening, you can strengthen up your make-up by adding a charcoal-colour eye shadow to the outer corners of the eyes, and perhaps a shadow with a slight glimmer or metallic fleck in it. There need not be a great deal of difference between your day and evening make-up, except perhaps a little sparkle on the eyes and lips.

2. Evening look

◇ Naturally, little can be done to change hair this short. However, a small amount of gel was used on the sides to give stronger emphasis to the lightness and natural movement of the top of her hair.

○ The whole eye area was lightly brushed with charcoal shadow, then a soft, pink-pearl powder was smudged on the outer corners of the eye. The same terracotta blusher was simply re-applied and a gold lip gloss was put over the existing lipstick to complement the overall warm, gold tones.

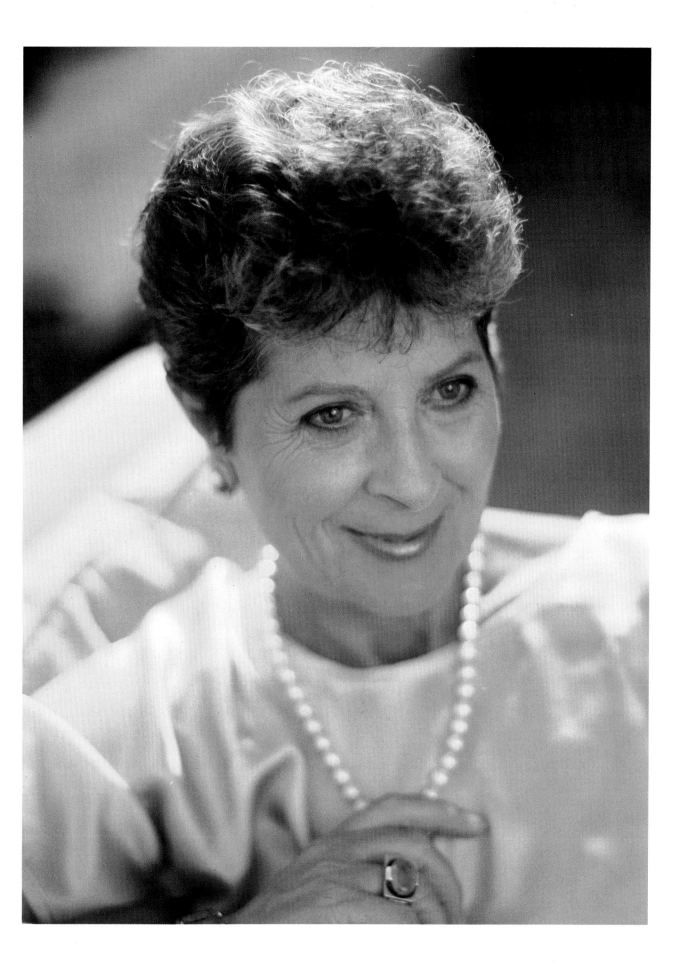

YOUNG PEOPLE

It is never too early to start looking after your skin. A thorough skin-care routine (cleansing, toning and moisturizing) begun at twelve or thirteen years old will set up a habit for life.

This is an age at which skin problems, such as spots, blackheads and acne may begin to appear. These reflect the normal hormonal changes taking place in your body which may occur at any time during the teenage years. Stress from examinations, important new relationships, the prospect of a career looming in the near future, and a tendency to eat 'junk food', often aggravate these skin problems. Junk food certainly plays a larger role than we like to believe. It is notoriously high in refined sugars, saturates, fats and salt, not to mention additives and preservatives, all of which have been proven beyond doubt to be harmful to the body and, therefore to the skin.

Proper diet, exercise, sleep and the right cleansing and moisturizing routine will help to keep your skin looking healthy. The right cleansing routine may include medicated products specially formulated for problem skin. However, if you are having serious skin problems you should consult a dermatologist or doctor.

○ Young skins are naturally beautiful. All the make-up you may need is a tinted moisturizer, a little mascara and a lip gloss or lipstick. If you have skin problems, you may want to hide your blemishes with a cover stick. You can use any colours you like, even vibrant ones, for eyes, lips and cheeks.

Make-up should really be fun! Enjoy it, experiment with it, and don't take it too seriously. If you don't like what you have done you can easily wash it off!

Remember that it is important to clean off your make-up before going to bed at night.

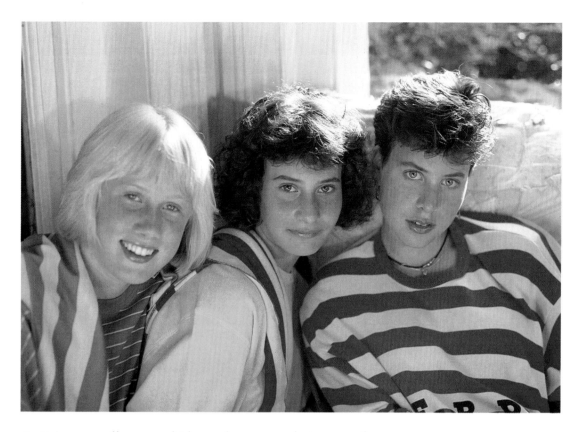

◇ It is generally a good idea to keep your hair away from your face so that it does not create, or aggravate skin problems. The styles here are simple, but do not inhibit the young person's natural inclination to experiment. Hair is a statement of independence which is part of the reason for the fantastic hair creations we see nowadays. Young people should be allowed to make mistakes as long as nothing is done to damage the hair, for example overprocessing it.

Chloe's hair (left) is very thick, very fair and very straight. It is cut in a graduated bob with a soft fringe to frame her face.

Natasha's hair (centre) is naturally curly. It has been cut in such a way that she can wash it, give it a shake, run her hands through it, and then forget about it.

Jessica's hair (right) is layered very close at the sides. Her hair is very thick and the natural bounce in it gives volume on top.

WEDDINGS

One of the most important questions that every bride will be asking is, 'How can I keep my hair looking beautiful throughout the whole of my wedding day?' There is so much activity and excitement surrounding a wedding that the last thing you want to worry about is your hair. It is wise to plan a hair-style that will look consistently good and last all day. You will find this more satisfying than creating a style that looks marvellous for a moment but collapses as soon as the ceremony is over.

It is best to look for the natural movement of the hair and to cut and style it to enhance this movement. This is preferable to trying to change the hair-style completely by making straight hair look curly or curly hair look straight, for example.

There are many variations on basic themes. For example, if you are a woman with shoulder-length, curly hair you might wear it up in a French pleat for the ceremony itself and then, in the evening, take it down and brush it softly through. Or, if you have short, straight hair cut in a bob then you could have a hair-piece tied into your hair for the wedding ceremony which could be plaited or bound with fresh flowers and ribbon. Then in the evening you could simply brush out your shiny short hair, allowing it to fall naturally around your face.

A wedding is a special occasion and it is essential to find the right fabrics and accessories to enhance the bride, match what she is wearing and also correspond with her own individual preferences and sense of occasion. It is a moment when the fragrance of fresh flowers placed in the hair can add a new dimension and create a beautifully subtle and delicate atmosphere.

Whatever accessory you decide to attach to the hair, make sure that it is not too heavy. If you want to be absolutely sure that the accessory is secure then grip it into the hair and sew it with thread; but make sure that you know how to cut it out again afterwards!

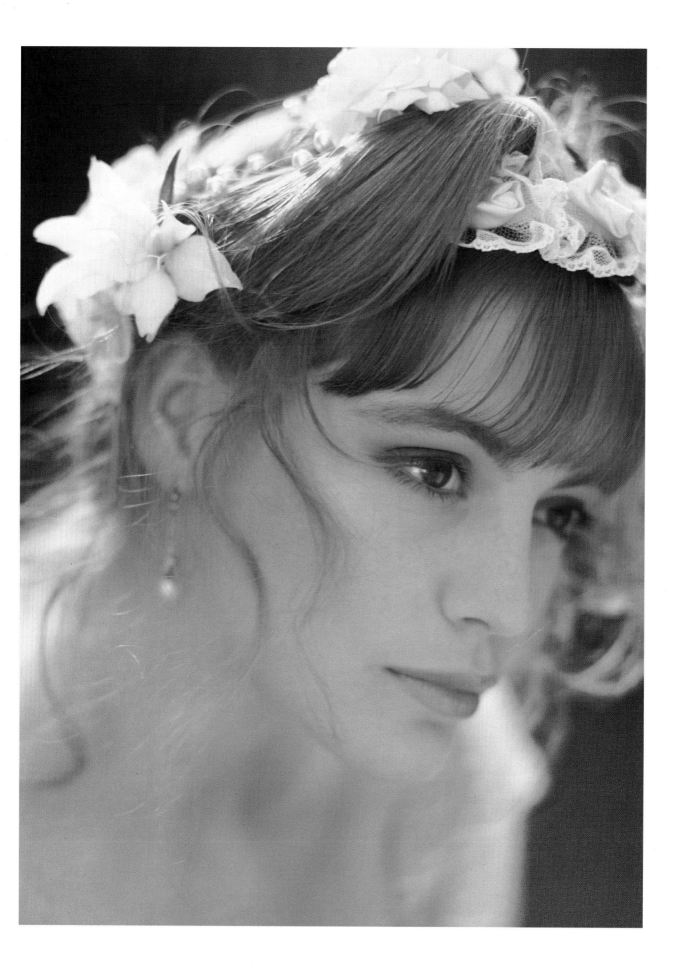

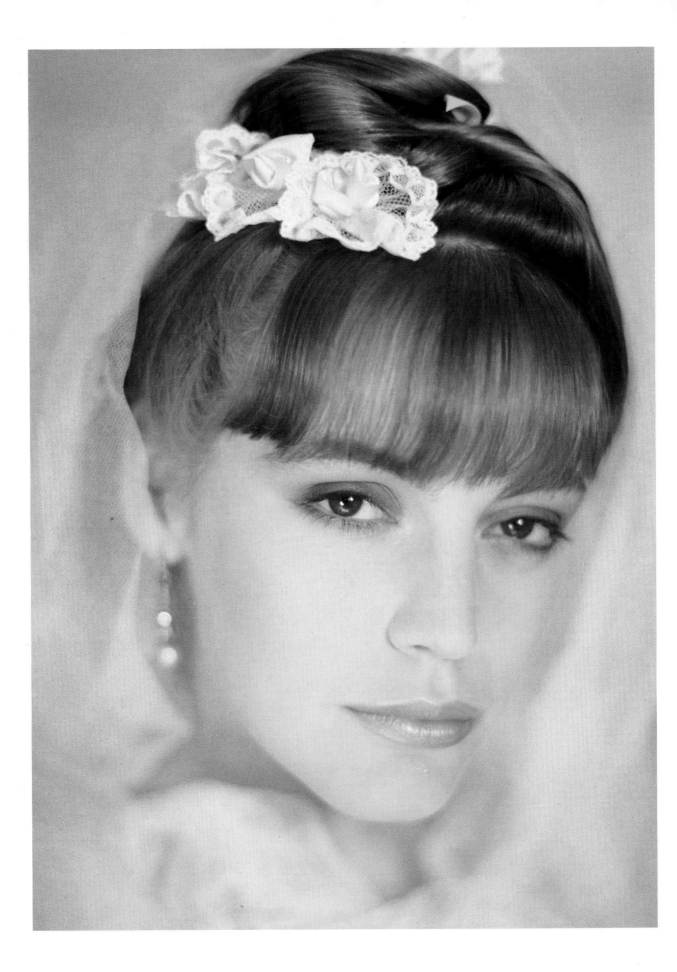

On this special day a woman looks for a balance between seriousness and sensuality. Her hair needs to be definite, but soft. The hair does not always need to be put up for a wedding but something should be placed in the hair to make it look more special than on any other day. When the hairdresser and the bride are working out what is to be done for the wedding, the hairdresser must incorporate the bride's own intuition about what she wants for the occasion.

It is essential that the hair goes right on the day so it is wise to have a trial run.

When deciding on make-up for a wedding, the bride will probably choose a soft, romantic look which allows her face to glow. In general, the shades most suitable for a wedding are soft, neutral tones which complement the natural colours of the skin, eyes and hair. I would use warm, earth tones on the eyes, and soft peaches and pinks on the lips.

◇ A light foundation matching the skin tone was put on the face and the eyebrows were brushed and shaped.

An apricot-colour eye shadow was brushed all over the eye area. Then a gold shadow was put on the lid and a copper-brown shadow was smudged on the outer corners and along the bottom lower lashes, to create a smoky effect. A red/bark mascara was used on the lashes, and a soft roses blusher enhanced the cheeks.

On the lips, a brown-pink lipstick was blotted and over the top we added touches of gold-flecked lip gloss.

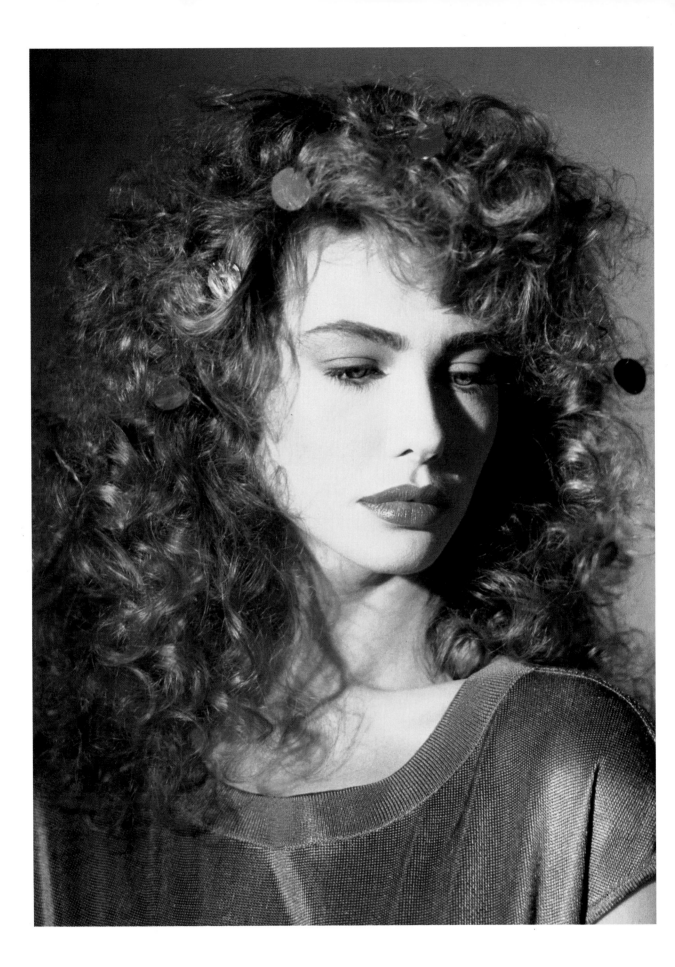

ANNA

◇ Anna's hair was towel and finger dried, set on Molton Browners, and left for forty-five minutes without any additional heat. Bronze, copper and silver sequins were then threaded through the hair to frame the face and pick up the colours of her dress and make-up.

○ The make-up has kept the overall feeling of colour in the clothes. There is a consistency in the hair and make-up which harmonizes with the subtlety of the colours and textures. The interest is in the hair, so the eyes are very simple and follow the same colours and tones as the dress and sequins.

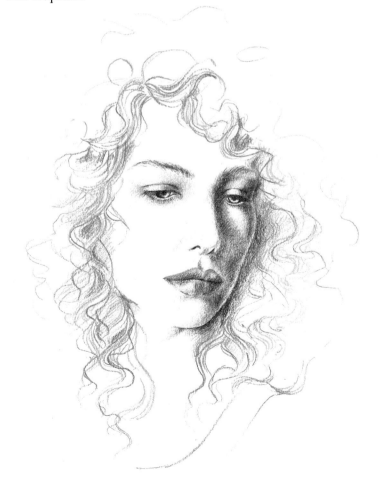

Foundation A beige foundation was put all over the face followed by a light dusting of translucent powder.

Eyes The eyebrows were shaped and brushed. The entire eyelid was brushed with an iridescent gold shadow. Then, raspberry iridescent was put on the upper lid and blended upwards to meet the gold. A brown eye liner was used on the upper lid and a bronze eye shadow was smudged over the top of it to create depth. The bronze shadow was also brushed underneath the lower lashes. A black mascara was put on both upper and lower lashes.

Cheeks A pale-raspberry shade of blusher was brushed over the cheeks.

Lips First the lips are covered with a rich, raspberry lipstick which is blotted. To finish, we applied a light covering of gold lip gloss which picks up the gold in the eyes and sequins.

a) Thread a sequin on to a needle threader.

b) Depending on the thickness of your hair, take five to ten strands and bend into a loop.

c) Pass the loop through the needle threader.

d) Pass the sequin from the needle threader on to the hair.

a)

b)

c)

d)

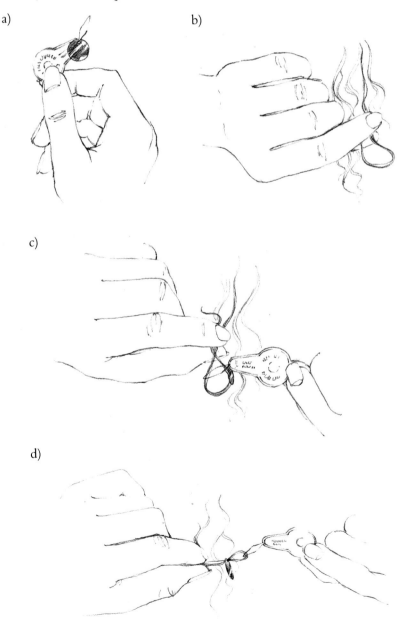

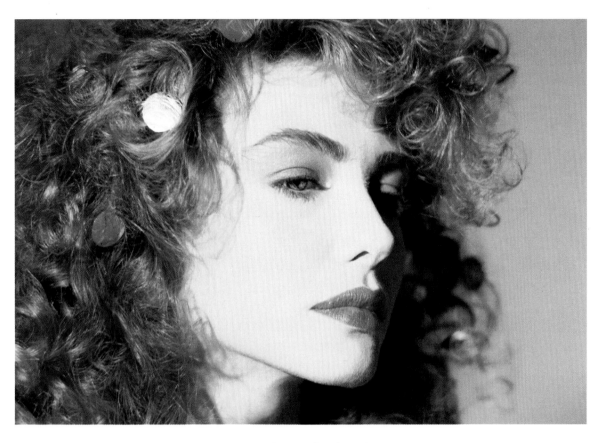

e) Pull the hair right through to free the needle threader.

f) Secure the sequin by knotting the end of the hair.

g) Leave the sequin to float in the hair.

e)   f)   g)

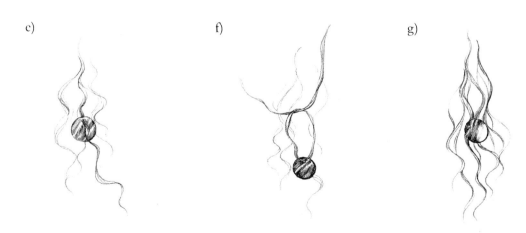

◇ Anna's hair, which is long, is set on Molton Browners and held in a pony tail to give the illusion of short hair.

○ Gold shimmer is the base eye shadow which was put all over the eye. Then a lilac shimmer was brushed — very lightly so that no line appeared — in the socket up to the bone of the eyebrow. A royal-blue eye shadow picks up the same colour in the beaded neck piece; this was used wet, as an eye liner, across the top of the lid. The lid was brushed with the same royal-blue eye shadow to soften the edge of the line. A black pencil was used under the lower lashes and in the very corner of the top lashes, then softened and smudged with a cotton bud. As a contrast, black mascara was put on the eyelashes. A lilac blusher was swept softly over the cheeks. Finally, to add sparkle to the lips, a lilac lipstick with a metallic fleck of silver glitter in it was used.

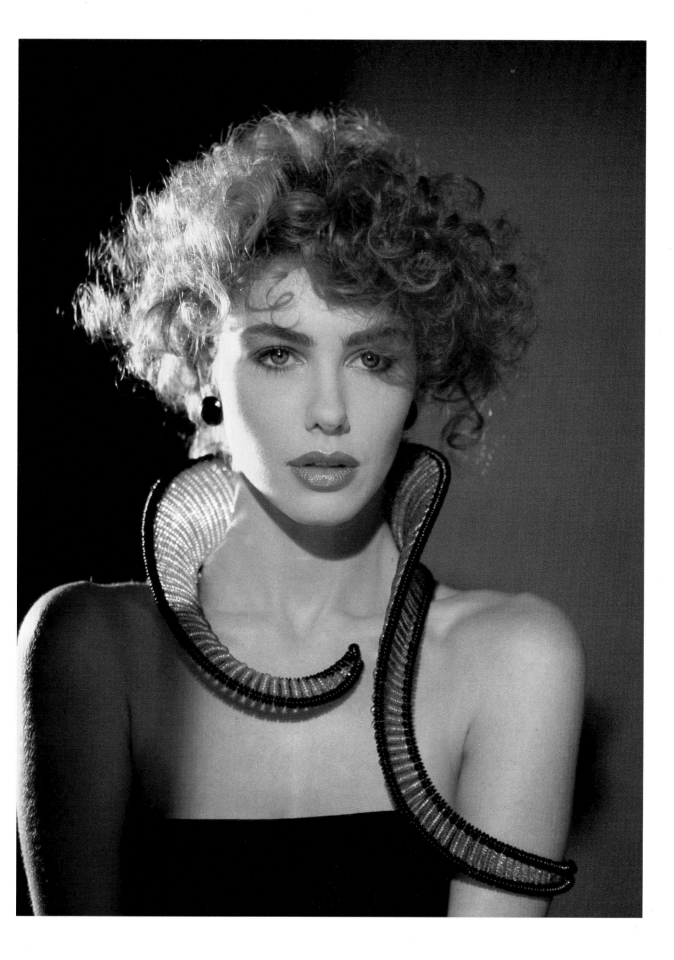

All of us who have been working on this book have been forced to look at our work in a fresh way, and this has had a two-fold effect. Firstly, we have had to re-affirm why we love to do our work. Secondly, it has made us realize how much more there is to learn. This has left us with a feeling of confidence and excitement for the future. This confidence and excitement is surely related to the essence of a woman's way of expressing herself — inwardly and outwardly — which we call *A Way of Looking*.

INDEX